Animals, Aging, and the Aged

THE
WESLEY W. SPINK
LECTURES ON
COMPARATIVE MEDICINE

Volume 5

ANIMALS, AGING, AND THE AGED

LEO K. BUSTAD

Dean, College of Veterinary Medicine
Washington State University
Pullman, Washington

UNIVERSITY OF MINNESOTA PRESS
Minneapolis

Published by the University of Minnesota Press,
2037 University Avenue Southeast, Minneapolis MN 55414
Printed in the United States of America

Library of Congress Cataloging in Publication Data

Bustad, Leo K
    Animals, aging, and the aged.
    (The Wesley W. Spink lectures on comparative
medicine; v. 5)
    A modified expansion of the 1979 lectures given
at the Duluth, Minneapolis, and St. Paul campuses of
the University of Minnesota.
    Bibliography: p.
    Includes index.
    1. Aging--Addresses, essays, lectures. 2. Aging--
Animal models--Addresses, essays, lectures.
3. Geriatrics--Addresses, essays, lectures. 4. Pets--
Psychological aspects--Addresses, essays, lectures.
I. Title. II. Series: Wesley W. Spink lectures on
comparative medicine; v. 5.
QP86.B83   612'.67'0724   80-24415
ISBN 0-8166-0977-7

The University of Minnesota
is an equal-opportunity
educator and employer.

The Wesley W. Spink Lectures on Comparative Medicine, established in honor of Dr. Spink's wide range of accomplishments, are presented by international authorities in comparative medicine and biology. A graduate of Carleton College and Harvard Medical School, Dr. Spink has maintained a deep interest in comparative medicine for almost forty years at the University of Minnesota, where he is now Regents' Professor Emeritus of Medicine and Comparative Medicine. Sponsorship of the lectures by the University of Minnesota reflects its concern for the dissemination of scientific knowledge. The lectures, and the publication of the volumes based on them, have been assisted by a grant from the Bush Foundation.

CONTENTS

LIST OF FIGURES

LIST OF TABLES

FOREWORD
Geriatric Education
and Training

The study of aging is not simply the study of decline and dysfunction or of disease and disability; it is the study of the normal processes of development. Because of the growing population in this country of people over 65—an estimated 31 million by the year 2000—the subject of aging is getting increased attention. We face a great challenge today, that of extending the active, creative, productive, and healthy middle years of the life cycle. To meet this challenge we must strive to change negative attitudes toward old age and overcome stereotypes many people have about the elderly; we must intensify our research efforts to acquire an understanding of the aging process and diseases associated with aging; and we must improve the social and economic conditions of older people.

Improved health-care technology is needed to reduce the financial burden of old age. In 1977 $10.5 billion was spent for nursing-home expenditures and $41.2 billion for all health-care expenditures for people over 65. Nursing-home admissions and health-care costs would drop dramatically if, for example, we had a better knowledge of the causes and treatment of osteoporosis, a thinning of the bones that leads to disabling hip fractures and frequently to institutionalization.

A greater understanding of age-related changes in response to drugs could prevent unnecessary falls and fractures caused by drug-induced dizziness and disorientation as well as transient confusion often misdiagnosed as "senility." By discovering the causes and developing more accurate diagnoses and effective treatment of organic brain disease we could greatly reduce the nursing-home population.

Animal studies have played a major role in helping us explore the mechanisms underlying the diseases prevalent in the later years. We have gained insight from animal investigations into the physiological changes with age. In this volume Dr. Bustad discusses another way in which animals can help older people: as companions for the elderly.

Medicine has a long way to go in effectively treating the diseases of old age. We have, however, begun to change our attitudes toward aging and the elderly. Research has brought us closer to understanding the aging process and improving geriatric care. This series of lectures by Dr. Bustad translates this body of knowledge into a readable and understandable form.

Robert N. Butler, M.D.

ACKNOWLEDGMENTS

Grateful acknowledgment is made for the helpful discussions with and input from: Marlene Adrian, Keith Banks, Bonnie Beaver, Douglas Bowden, John Brunzell, Gary Bryan, Leo B. Bustad, Clarence Chrisp, Tom Clarkson, Sam Corson, Jean Dodds, Caleb Finch, Michael Fox, John Glomset, Marvin Goldman, Gilbert Gordan, Don Gibson, Tom Griggs, Joe Held, Carol Hollander, Glenn Horstman, Webster Jee, Mark Hegsted, Tom Kawakami, Charles Leathers, Edward Masoro, Joe Mauderly, Roger McClellan, Ed Menning, Ken Meyers, Richard Ott, Lance Perryman, David Prieur, Kathy Quinn, Fred Rapp, Sue Ritter, Terry Ryan, George Sacher, Howard Schneider, Fred Smithcors, Bill Spangler, Leon Rosenblatt, Kaia Sorem, Richard Torbeck, Marshall Urist, Robert Wilson, and Leon Whitney and Tom Wolfle.

Special thanks are extended to my wife, Signe, for her support and bibliographic work, Linda Hines for her heroic and outstanding efforts in editing, Vicki Croft and associates in the Health Sciences Library, Marie Zeglen and associates in Biomedical Communications for their excellent productions in the graphic arts (also used for the lectures), my administrative assistant, Joyce Schafer, for helpful support in many areas, Michele Sebti and Steve Cox for their outstanding efforts in entering rough manuscripts onto computer datasets, and Alan Hagen-Wittbecker for producing a readable manuscript.

The good that is in this book is a credit to those listed above and in the bibliography. The responsibility for errors is mine.

Leo K. Bustad
Washington State University

INTRODUCTION

This book is a modified expansion of the 1979 Wesley Spink lectures given at the Duluth, Minneapolis, and St. Paul campuses of the University of Minnesota on Animal Contributions to Understanding Aging, Geriatric Medicine, and The Elderly.

Unfortunately, most definitions and descriptions of aging carry negative connotations. Webster's Seventh New Collegiate Dictionary (1961) defines aging as "to become old, to show or impart the characteristics of increasing age as weakness, maturity, or crystalline or chemical change." Shakespeare's words in *As You Like It* are more poignant, and certainly more negative:

Last scene of all,
That ends this strange eventful history,
Is second childishness and mere oblivion,
Sans teeth, sans eyes, sans taste, sans every thing.
[2. 7. 163-169]

This bleak image has plagued me since I first committed it to memory at the age of fourteen.

My definition, I believe, is more realistic, definitely more optimistic. *Aging is the process associated with attaining maturity. After mid-adulthood it is characterized by a variable decrease in viability and by increases in vulnerability, wisdom, and appreciation for each day.* I intend to pursue vigorously the means for eliminating, or at least diminishing, some of the disagreeable changes that accompany aging. I seek to optimize our biological potential for both mind and body as we grow older.

If I were to select one word to describe my purpose in these lectures, it would be *heart* — in its many connotations. I've tried to review the "heart" of the genuine concerns about aging that old people have expressed to me over many years. I've tried to get to the "heart" of the disease problems such as cardiovascular disease and cancer, which concern so many people. I've tried to summarize many of the factors that will make our hearts work better and longer, for the failure of this muscle causes our greatest mortality. And I've tried to show "heart," that is, concern for all who would benefit by "feeling heart" animal companions, since I firmly believe that a properly selected and trained animal can help us feel better and can even make our hearts beat longer and more effectively. Perhaps animals help because of what George McDonald (Lewis, 1949) observed in his *Sir Gibbie:*

The bliss of the animals lies in this fact, that on their lower level, they shadow the bliss of those. . . . who do not "look before and after, and pine for what is not" but live in the holy carelessness of the eternal now.

From them we may learn this secret, of "living in the holy carelessness of the eternal now."

The subjects I have chosen to discuss are those for which considerable data are available, those of special interest to me, and those subjects that can be profitably addressed experimentally. Furthermore, even the present knowledge in some of these areas can assist both the old and those who hope to grow old.

Animals have been used in answering some questions of major concern to old people, as reflected in their conversations with me over a number of years. In planning this book,

I deliberately addressed issues of great concern in my own life and in the lives of my older associates, friends and strangers, emphasizing those conditions with a significant nutritional component. Some of the questions posed to me were:

- What causes aging?
- Is it true that when you stop growing you start dying?
- What diseases will most probably "get" me, and can I prevent some of them?
- How should I keep fit?
- Is exercise a good thing and, if so, how much?
- Do we need more sleep when we get old?
- Is there anything I can do about the loss of taste and smell?
- What should I eat?
- Should I eat fewer calories, less protein and sugar?
- Does high sugar intake really cause diabetes?
- What about fats? Some tell us to use polyunsaturates, yet other reports say they may cause cancer and increased cholesterol in the blood. What should we believe?
- Should I take extra vitamins and minerals?
- Should I consume a lot of fiber, and does eating more fiber change my requirements for other dietary components?
- Can one prevent senility?
- Loss of mental ability and loneliness are what I fear most: What can I do about them?
- Is most of what happens to us in old age determined when we are young, or is it all determined genetically?

This volume explores where and how animals have contributed significantly to understanding aging and to helping the aged. In view of the broad scope of the topic, I will concentrate on how animals used in life span studies can answer many of the questions the elderly are asking and to which they deserve answers.

Chapter 1 provides a perspective on animals and the ways they have assisted mankind from earliest recorded history.

In Chapter 2, I discuss what we have learned from animals about what happens to them as they age. The extent to which these changes in animals resemble what happens in people will also be discussed.

Chapter 3 focuses on knowledge gained from animal studies that can assist old people and those who provide for the health and well-being of the elderly. Cardiovascular disease and cancer, with brief mention of osteoporosis, periodontal disease, and age-related mental conditions, and how our life style, especially our diet, may modify these chronic degenerative diseases are the principal concerns in this chapter.

In the last chapter (4), I explore the role of companion animals in contributing to the physical and psychological well-being of our aging population. A first attempt is made to develop criteria of selection for animal placement to furnish a reference base for more definitive studies and evaluation. This last chapter is by necessity more anecdotal, since few systematic studies are available, but this should not detract from its validity.

In view of the breadth of subjects covered, I have been necessarily selective in the material reviewed. However, my concern has been to present the latest information available. When I did not have first-hand knowledge of a subject and could not find recent data, I spoke directly with a recognized authority or someone conducting relevant research in the field.

In the *Afterword,* I have summarized what I consider the critical issues and needs, gleaned from what we have learned about the elderly. This information could be useful for our youth as they look ahead to more healthful and rewarding old age. It is my sincere hope that the issues I address in this book will help not only the elderly, but those who are young and in between.

Animals, Aging, and the Aged

PERSPECTIVES ON ANIMALS

*The health of a people and their animals is really the founda-
tion upon which their happiness and their powers as a state
depend.*

Benjamin Disraeli

In 1855, Chief Sealth of the Duwamish Tribe in my home
state of Washington wrote a letter to the president of the
United States. His letter contained a great truth:

What is a man without beasts? If all the beasts were gone, men would die
from great loneliness of spirit, for whatever happens to the beast also
happens to man. All things are connected. Whatever befalls the earth befalls the sons of the earth. (Rynearson, 1978)

Having spent most of my scientific career in the field of
comparative medicine, I am continually reminded of people's
relationship to nonhuman life in the environment. Comparative medicine should be defined broadly as the study of the
nature, cause, and cure of abnormal structure and function in
people, animals, and plants for the eventual application to, and
the benefit of, all living things (Bustad, et al., 1976). "Function" is used here in a comprehensive sense that includes behavior, particularly the ways in which animals help us understand psychological abnormalities, as well as prevent and treat
abnormalities (Mugford and M'Comisky, 1975). However,
this definition does not restrict us to a one-way exchange of

3

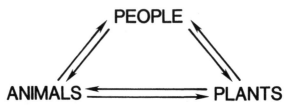

Figure 1. Comparative medicine is the study of the
nature, cause, and cure of abnormal structure and
function in people, animals, and plants for the eventual application to and benefit of all living things.

benefits from animals to people. Instead, benefits move back
and forth between people and animals, people and plants, and
animals and plants (Figure 1).

Plants and animals in our environment are like parts of our
body; If we eliminate them, we destroy part of ourselves. People must remain in contact with and relate to the environment
throughout their lifetime to remain healthy. A strong people-
animal-plant bond is critical to a healthy community.

Having been raised on a farm with animals, plants, and forests, I cannot imagine being separated from these elements of
our habitat. As a member of my high school's animal and plant
judging teams, I visited mental hospitals, reform schools, and
retirement homes, institutions which at that time included
farms with animals and plants. Much later I observed the effects of the loss of these farms when my own father entered a
retirement home. For cost-benefit risk reasons, animals were
banned at many institutions. As a result, old people were separated from animals at a time when the animals might be the
only source of continual, unconditional love, comfort, and
companionship.

History provides valuable insight into people-pet interactions. In earlier times, when more wisdom seemed to prevail,
people were treated in "Schweitzerian" fashion. The family,
including the animals, were part of the healing team. Often
the animals provided succor and warmth to ill persons and
contributed to their well-being. Throughout recorded history,

even in prehistoric times, people and animals lived together. Animals played a significant role in human customs, legends, and religions (Barloy, 1974). For example, recall the importance of the cat in ancient Egypt. Many civilizations have been, and continue to be, shaped by economic dependence on animals—reindeer, caribou, llamas, sheep, and goats.

Animals once lived in close proximity to people, often occupying the same quarters (a practice that continues today in many regions). Barloy (1974) recalls in certain regions in France that cattle and pigs lived on the ground floor of a dwelling place while the family, poultry, and piglets occupied the first floor. Children and animals crawled together on the floor. Sometimes goats and sheep slept beside members of the family. In some alpine areas, people huddled together with animals for up to six months of the year, and the dung would accumulate until spring. In my youth, it was not unusual for farmers to bring sick animals into the house so that they could minister to the animals all night. In Africa, Normandy, Sicily, and other places, residents adorn some animals with ornaments and tufts of colored wool. It is more common in our age to adorn automobiles instead of animals, and psychologically we are the poorer for it.

A lonely dilemma descends upon a people when they are separated from the elemental processes of nature, for we are parts of one interdependent and remarkable community. Early in our history, we identified intimately with both inanimate and animate elements of our surroundings. Some of the first drawings and paintings depicted people with animals. There is every indication that people adopted pets or animals not only as helpers, but as companions.

Primitive people found that people-animal partnerships were important to their well-being, if not vital to their survival. Many of earth's early inhabitants formed a strong alliance, even a symbiotic relationship, with animals. The most noteworthy relationship was with the dog. Perhaps the very first was man and dog hunting together in a mutual assistance pact. Through the process of domestication, each became dependent on the other, and evenually probably neither could have survived alone. Undoubtedly, it would have been far more difficult for man to hunt other animals for food without the dog's scent-tracking and attack capabilities. Other animals, too, helped people secure food and the bare necessities of life.

One of the most fascinating partnerships involves dolphins. This relationship was first described by Pliny the Elder in the first century A.D., but it was not believed. More recently, Professor Rene-Guy Busnel reported his discoveries on the Mauritanian coast (Barloy, 1974). There, local fishermen checked the color of the sea for the approach of a shoal of mullet. As soon as they sighted the shoal, a man entered the water and beat vigorously with a stick. Within minutes the dolphins were alerted and usually came in packs of ten. The fishermen put out their nets so that the mullet were cornered, and the dolphins drove them into the nets. Through teamwork fishing, man and dolphins got some of the "take." Pliny's early account of the dolphin along the coast of the Lanquedoc region was essentially the same as the more recent report.

Another unusual symbiotic relationship exists with the honey guide. A bird about the size of a starling, the honey guide is very fond of bee larvae and bee's wax, which it is unable to obtain because of a weak beak. Upon discovering a wild honey tree, the bird will seek out a honey badger or ratel (an African beast of prey) and lead it to the newly discovered beehive. The badger with its large claws is able to provide access to the bee brood and the bee's wax. The thick skin of the badger protects it from bee stings. In the absence of a badger, the indicator bird will seek out a person to lead to the honey. Many of the natives in the bird's place of residence have accepted this cooperation between two individuals of different species (Barloy, 1974). Through such associations a strong kinship and mutual respect developed between people and animals that has been perpetuated by many enlightened people to this day.

It is noteworthy that early people often worshiped or recognized beasts as special. They looked at animals as possessing cunning, courage, healing potential, and power beyond their own. Animals, like people, were animated by a soul, and could continue beyond death. Since they thought these beasts understood human language, they communicated with them. Early people talked very seriously to animals and asked pardon when it was their painful duty to hunt and kill them. The North American Indian would reason with a horse as if it were rational.

The sense of an absolute distinction or separation between man and beast so prevalent in our world was hardly to be found among the early dwellers of our earth. Indians in Eastern Washington told in their oral literature about the time of the Animal World, when animals of today were supposed to be in the intermediate stage between man and animal. They resembled humans, but were able to turn themselves into animals at will, as the old Indian doctors were believed to do. The tales recount the exploits of frog woman (Figure 2), salmon man, owl woman, and others. The demi-god Coyote was actually the ancestor of the Indians in the tales. For a time animals and people combined to rule the world. Eventually the generations of man came to stay and animals chose their permanent beastly form. But the Great Spirit gave Indians His special powers through the medium of animals. For example, the greatest hunters received special power from the animal being hunted, such as the deer (Hines, 1976).

The history of the development of the use of animals as "therapeutic facilitators" for improving the health and well-bing of people is an interesting one. Summarized below, the history is admittedly sparse in systematic, studied approach and written documentation.

Early Accounts

It is impossible to determine when animals were first used to promote the physical and psychological well-being of people. Recent evidence suggests that dogs were companions for man possibly even before their use in hunting or as guardians (Davis and Valla, 1978; Messent, 1979). The evidence consists of a fossil skeleton of a man, believed to be from 12,000 B.C., with his hand resting on a young dog. This Israeli find coincided

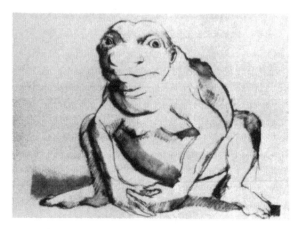

Figure 2. Frog Woman: a character in the oral literature of the Okanogan tribe.

with a similar find of the same dating in Iraq. Recent excava-
tions along the Yukon's Old Crow River in North America led
by Drs. William Irving and Brenda Beebe have turned up jaws
of several domesticated dogs at least 30,000 years old, almost
20,000 years older than any other known domesticated animal (Canby, 1979). These dogs may have served as readily
available sources of protein to the domesticators, as well as
being companions or hunters.

One of the famous dogs of ancient literature was Argus,
who lay dying as Odysseus returned from Troy after twenty
years of wandering. Argus wagged his tail and dropped his ears,
he alone recognizing his old master. In Aristophanes' play
"Wasps," the hero's father is in his second childhood and has
to be shut in to keep from sitting in the law courts. The old
man spends his days playing court, with the dog playing the
part of the accused.

Animals and parts of animals were in the armamentarium
of medicine men throughout history. The pharmacopoeia of
almost every nation referred to the use of various parts of certain animals in therapy (Levinson, 1969a). The cat was thought

by many ancients to possess supernatural powers (Hall and Browne, 1904). Some remarkable preventive and therapeutic measures for an assortment of conditions included:

- Erysipelas: Cut off the ear of a cat and let the blood drip on the affected part
- Whitlow: Place affected finger in the ear of a cat for 15 minutes each day
- Epilepsy and lameness: Use fat from a wild cat
- Prevention of blindness: Blow ashes from the burnt head of a black cat into the eyes three times each day.

Dogs, too, occupied an esteemed place on the healing team. Dogs were used to lick patients to promote healing in ancient Greece (Halliday, 1922) since healing properties were attributed to the dog's tongue. A French proverb runs, "Langue de chien, sert de medicine" (The dog's tongue serves as medicine). Dogs were closely associated with Asclepius, the god of healing. Even today, in Turkana dogs serve as "nurses" to clean up babies' vomit and excrement (Schwabe, 1978).

Pliny thought that stomach pains could be healed by transfering them to a pup. In Philemon Holland's sixteenth century translation of Pliny's *Naturall Historie*, he credited Pliny with this sage advice regarding lap dogs: "The pretty little dogs that our daintie dames make so much of, if they be ever and anon kept close unto the stomacke, they ease the pain thereof." The sixteenth century physician John Keyes echoed this sentiment with words about lap dogs being good to "assuage the sickness of the stomacke, being oftimes thereunto applied as a plaster preservative." He also stated these "delicate, neate, and pretty kind of Dogges called the spaniel-gentle, or comforter," were sought for by "daintie dames." These dogs were often wet-nursed by "ordinary men's wives" for "ladies of quality" (Smithcors, 1959). In very early times, too, if a person felt in danger of going insane, he would carry a dog about with him. Evidence indicates that this works in a somewhat different context today, as will be discussed in Chapter 4 and is receiving much current attention (Lorenz, 1953; Herriot, 1977; Hesketh, 1978).

Our regard for animals is reflected even in our laws. America is credited as the first country to put humane laws regarding animals into writing. In 1641, the Puritans of the Massachusetts Bay Colony established "The Body of Liberties." "Liberty" 92 read: "No man shall exercise any Tirrany or Crueltie towards any bruite creature . . . kept for man's use" (Leavitt, 1968). Obviously, animals were viewed as property, to be used, but not unnecessarily abused. In 1828, New York became the first state to adopt anticruelty legislation. In 1866, Henry Bergh incorporated the country's first humane society, the American Society for the Prevention of Cruelty to Animals (ASPCA) to actively enforce the existing laws of the day.

Animals have become very popular in our day, sometimes for different reasons than in the past. In cities where little association with nature exists, a dog, cat, canary, or goldfish give a glimpse of the natural world. The number of companion animals has increased remarkably. Estimates show there are approximately 70 million dogs and cats in this country (Carding, 1975; Wilbur, 1976; Wallin, 1978; Friedmann, et al., 1979). Also, many of the eight or nine million horses are companion animals. Add to this list countless birds, goats, rabbits, guinea pigs, hamsters, gerbils, fish, pigs, and a wide assortment of "creepy-crawlies," and we probably end up with an average of at least one companion animal for every man, woman, and child in America. The Wilbur (1976) survey indicated that 55% of the households in the United States had a dog or cat or both. Even the number of birds is increasing remarkably. In a recent survey conducted in a section of a large western city, more than half of the homes had at least one bird (West, personal communication, 1979). A comparison of the number of homes having pets in several countries in Europe and the United States appears in Table 1.

The importance of the people-pet bond, which includes using animals as companions and therapists, finally seems to be generally recognized and action based on that knowledge will become more common in the near future (Fogle, 1979; see Hediger, 1965; McCulloch, 1976, 1977, 1979). Recent data

Table 1. Percentage of Homes in Various Countries
Having One or More Pets

| | Kind of Animal | | |
Country	Dogs	Cats	Birds
Belgium	22	21	23
Britain	27	18	14
Denmark	25		
France	29	25	14
Finland		28	1
Germany	9	9	13
Ireland	45	38	
Italy	19	23	
Netherlands			21
Portugal		28	
Spain			12
United States	33	12	20

(10% homes in U.S. had both cats and dogs; total = 55%.)

(Barloy, 1974; McCulloch, 1976; Wilbur, 1976.)

suggest that companion animals will often encourage improved self-care in their owners, including better nutrition, and will contribute to their owners' remaining independent longer (Corson, et al., 1975, 1979). Animals also can be a source of great comfort to the ill and lonely and may well promote the well-being and prolong the lives of heart attack victims (Friedmann, et al., 1979). Animal-facilitated therapy regimes may be in some cases equally as important as animals' use in developing new surgical procedures, and in certain cancer and nutrition research.

CHAPTER 2

ANIMAL CONTRIBUTIONS TO UNDERSTANDING AGING

The sixth age shifts
Into the lean and slipper'd pantaloon.
With spectacles on nose and pouch on side,
His youthful hose, well savd, a world too wide
For his shrunk shank; and his manly voice,
Turning again toward childish treble, pipes
And whistles in his sound.
[As You Like It, 2. 7. 156-162]

The process of aging in people has long captured the imagination of our poets and challenged our scientists. Insight into this process has been provided by many species of animals that I have observed for their entire life span. Everyone at one time or another, if only to oneself, asks: "How long can I expect to live?" People also ask about the life span of their animals (see Table 2). Among the animals I've studied, the laboratory mice and rats never reached four years of age. Our oldest dog approached 18, as did our oldest cat, and our miniature pigs seemed to have similar survival curves. We had cows that were 17 years old. Although few cows reach 20, I received a picture of a man and his pet Jersey cow, which he said was 32 years old when it died. We have had horses over 30 years old, but have heard reports of some as old as 50. Higher primates have been known to live over 30 years. The oldest mammals other than man are elephants, which have been reported to live over 70 years, an age comparable to that of many people. Maximum life spans in animals, especially long-lived ani-

12

Table 2. Comparative Chronological Ages of People and Animals

	People	Pig	Dog	Horse	Mouse
	100	17	20	50	3 Yrs.
	90	15	18	45	
	80	13	16	40	
Wise			15		
	70	11	14	35	2-2½
		10	13		
	60	9	11		
		8	10		
	50	7	8	25	
Middle		6	7		1½
	40	5	6	20	
		4	5		
	30	3	4	10	
Adult		2	2		
	20			4	4-6 Mos.
Youth		0.6	1	2	
	10			1.5	6 Wks.

Adapted from Lebeau, 1970, for dog; and personal communications from Horstman, Gillis, and Ragan, 1979, for pig; Torbeck, 1979, for horse; and Sacher, 1979, for mouse.

mals, are as difficult to determine as those of people and for much the same reasons—inadequate records, poor memories, or prevarication on the part of the owners.

A person who has lived an active life well in excess of 100 years, even to 120, or who has an animal that has lived an unusually long life, is considered newsworthy. Several areas in the world are famous for having very long-lived people. Often-mentioned regions are the Ecuadorian Andes, the western Himalayas in northern Kashmir, and the Caucasus Mountains in southern Russia. The few people who live in these regions have many common characteristics, including life in a remote region, a high illiteracy rate, a life of hard physical labor, and limited nutrition relative to the intake of fats, proteins, and calories. They also have poor birth records, poor memories, and probably lie about their age.

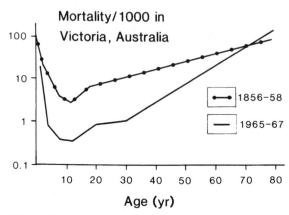

Figure 3. Mortality data for 1856-58 compared with
that for 1965-67 in Melbourne, Australia
(Burnet, 1974).

We really have not extended the maximum life span of
animals appreciably, nor have we extended our own maximum life span of about 115 in several millennia. What we
have done is control infectious diseases in much of the world,
permitting more animals to reach their full potential and
more people to reach the Biblical three score and ten (Siegal,
1975). Few people have worked harder in studying and controlling these infectious diseases than Wesley Spink, whom
we honor with these lectures (Spink, 1979).

Expression

It is useful to express life span and mortality data graphically.
The best known curves for plotting mortality and survival
data are the Gompertz plot and a curve expressing the percent survivors as a function of age (Jones, 1956; Sacher,
1956, 1977; and see Blumenthal, 1978). The Gompertz
plot, since it was first presented in 1825, has had a universal
application expressing the "force of mortality" for mammals
and many other species. As first used, it represented a com-
posite of deaths associated with disease. If we plot age-
related mortality rates for various diseases discussed in this

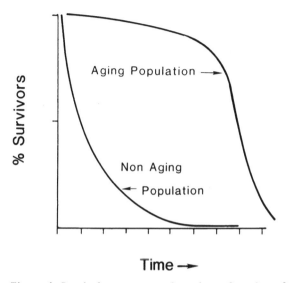

Figure 4. Survival percentage plotted as a function of age. In one case the curve shows 50% survival at each time period (and resembles that of wolfhounds, for unexplained reasons) (Comfort, 1956); in the other, the typical survival curve of an aging population (such as beagles or people).

book, such as cancer and coronary heart disease, a straight line relationship is obtained that varies only slightly in slope on a Gompertzian plot. Burnet (1974) used a Gompertz plot to show that optimal survival occurs through the period of maximum reproductive capacity (about 15-30 years of age for people). This period of life benefits from maximum efficiency of the immune and neuroendocrine systems (see Figure 3).

Probably the most commonly used method is to plot survivors as a function of age. As diseases and mortality of the young have been controlled, the curve has become more rectangular, which characterizes a typical aging population, such as beagles or people, in the Western world and contrasts with animals that incur the same percentage of deaths throughout life (Figure 4). Strangely, Irish wolfhounds also show this latter type of mortality curve (Comfort, 1956).

Mortality data on most domestic animals (other than rodents) is limited. Some of the most dependable data are on thoroughbred horses in the United Kingdom (Comfort, 1956) and on beagle dogs from United States laboratories. With regard to the latter, it is interesting to note that dogs kept in outside runs at the University of California-Davis had an average life span of over 12 years, whereas some of their littermates placed in good homes as pups had an average survival rate of less than 5 years, principally owing to accidents.

Patterns of Aging

In observing many animals, including sheep, goats, swine, cattle, horses, dogs, chickens, rats, and mice, for a life span, I have noted that individuals in each species exhibited different patterns of aging. Few died on the same day in the same way, and no specific organ system consistently failed. Even highly inbred mice seemed to show varying patterns of aging. However, certain inbred strains manifested a very high incidence of certain diseases (for example, mammary cancer, renal disease, lymphoma), suggesting a significant genetic component in the aging process. On the other hand, aging mammals have many characteristics in common, including a gradual reduction in the immune response, a reduced output of certain hormones, an increase in the incidence of tumors, and a host of anatomical and physiological changes. As scientists observed and described these changes, many of them speculated (sometimes on rather limited evidence) that the specific aging changes they observed were the bases for the general events observed in the aging individual. Based on these observations, a host of hypotheses and aging theories were proposed.

Twenty years ago, while preparing my Ph.D. thesis at the University of Washington School of Medicine, I reviewed many of the reports on aging changes and the most prominent theories then discussed, which were developed to explain the anatomical and physiological changes observed in aging and to explain aging itself.

As I noted in 1960, the anatomical and physiological changes observed with aging in higher animals include organ atrophy; reduction in the cellularity of the central nervous system; increase in the amount of fat, connective tissue, and cellular pigment; decrease in muscular strength, reaction time, fertility, oxygen utilization, and cardiac output; deterioration of vision and hearing; reduced adaptability to environmental changes; slower recovery rate following injury; and change in the concentrations of chemical constituents, including an increase in sulfur, calcium, and sodium, and a decrease in potassium (Bustad, 1960).

I noted then that the contribution made to general senescence by aging cells of specific organs was not fully defined, but it appeared that no one organ represented the limiting case. Rather, the processes of aging seemed to be fairly general with regard to various organs. The change in the stem cells seemed to be a progressive one that affected the quality of the regenerating cells; the life of the nondividing cells, although fixed, was subject to reduction by injury and passage of time.

Since writing my thesis, I have observed many animals over their life span. As a physiologist I am impressed that most components of the internal environment of mammals are maintained at fairly normal levels under resting, steady-state conditions even into advanced age (Goldstein and Reichel, 1978; Kohn, 1977; Masoro, 1979; Shock, 1974, 1977, 1979; Timiras, 1978). Animals and people do share a common loss of physiological efficiency with advancing age that becomes obvious when they are "put to the test." One can observe and recall the young of all species in their play. They seem to be able to run, jump, and climb all day. The young of all species seem to be characterized by a substantial redundancy in physiological capacity, with a considerable reserve. This redundancy and reserve seem to diminish with time, with the death or dysfunction of many, but not all, cells and tissues.

Age-related changes are quite noticeable in the appearance of many animals, especially dogs, nonhuman primates, and most people—the greying and thinning of hair; the wrinkled skin; the slowing, less steady gait; the loss of acuity in vision and audition. It is obvious that the form of youth is modified; some parts of the body may appear somewhat flabby and fat. People more than animals seem to grow, as my father said, "like a cow's tail—downward." The skeleton becomes smaller, and people become shorter. Problems with the teeth occur, and these changes are usually obvious. Other changes are less obvious to the eye. The capacity to adjust to one's surroundings is considerably diminished; healing is somewhat impaired. Efficiency and speed are reduced. The cardiovascular changes include an increase in systolic blood pressure, and in the resistance of the blood vessels, which can be related to atherosclerosis. The heart rate is reduced, as is the amount of blood pumped by the heart each minute and the ability of the arteries to stretch. The work of the heart per stroke volume is increased. As for lung function, the vital capacity (the volume of gas that can be expelled from the lungs after a full inspiration) and the maximum breathing capacity (the measure of the lungs while breathing for fifteen seconds as deeply and as fast as possible), along with the partial pressure of oxygen, are reduced whereas the peripheral airway resistance and the dead space are increased. The senses of smell and taste are also diminished. The reduction in total capacity and oxygen consumption all contribute to diminished metabolic rate. Kidney function also is affected in the elderly, with the reduced renal blood flow, glomerular filtration rate, and the ability for concentration and dilution.

The age when various functional and structural changes occur varies greatly. Many people regard old age as something that begins at their sixty-fifth birthday; some argue that the designated time should be changed to seventy, and others suggest thirty. Very little substantial biological data, however, support the contention that people lose competency at 65 or 70. Most of the selected losses of performance can be easily accommodated in our society if we genuinely wish to take advantage of the unique capabilities and wisdom of the elderly.

Physiological Changes

One difficulty in discussing physiological changes of advancing age lies in separating normal from abnormal changes. What may be normal for one age could be abnormal for another. Too many studies have been performed on old, ill animals or people and the resulting observations reported as normal values for a given age. Similarly, cross-sectional studies have examined physiological functions at one point in time for individuals of varying ages, to establish criteria for physiological age, rather than studying a given species for a generation (that is, longitudinally, from birth to death) (Bustad et al., 1968; Bustad, 1970).

The following discussion of physiological changes with advancing age emphasizes those changes that might be subject to modification by feasible means of assisting the elderly. Structural and functional changes do not suddenly become manifest in old age, but begin at conception. Perceptible functional decrements in many systems can be described, not after 60 years, but usually with 30 years as a starting point, as shown in Figure 5.

One might regard Figure 5 as a preliminary step toward developing a physiological aging chart. Obviously, far more data on longitudinal studies are needed to have the equivalent of a growth chart for the young of a species, but such a chart would be worthwhile. It is important to realize that the decline in the various functions is not always linear. For example, vision begins failing in young adults and usually reaches a minimum by about age 50; hearing begins a gradual decline from adolescence to age 50, after which the rate of decline slows. The nature and age of decline depends a great deal on the experience of the individual. Loud noises early in life,

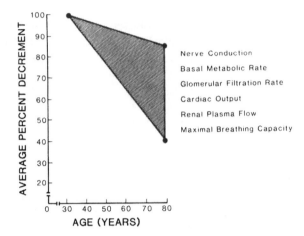

Figure 5. Age-related changes in some physiologic functions (ages 30-80). The various functions are listed in the order of the least change, observed in the nerve conduction, to the greatest change, observed in maximal breathing capacity. This latter capacity is in contrast to the vital capacity, and is less marked (modified from Shock, 1962, 1977; Masoro, 1976; Masoro et al., 1979).

for example, some contemporary music, can cause an earlier and greater decrement, while a relatively noise-free environment, as in certain African areas, can delay decrement somewhat (Timiras, 1978).

Cardiovascular Function

Leonardo da Vinci, on the basis of his dissections, believed that the cause of aging was

veins which by the thickening of their tunics in the old restrict the passage of blood, and by this lack of nourishment destroy the life of the aged without any fever, the old coming to fail little by little in slow death. (Belt, 1952)

Others have expressed the view that we are as old as our arteries. The heart and arteries have appropriately received much attention (Kohn, 1977). The heart rate generally slows from adulthood to old age; the diastolic pressure gradually increases while the systolic pressure changes little until old age, when it may increase markedly (Masoro et al., 1979). The cardiac output (the amount of blood pumped by the heart at rest) declines with age. In people, it declines at a rate of about one percent per year after ages 20-30.

The ability of the arteries to distend or stretch under pressure is reduced with age. This occurs independently of atherosclerosis, which can also affect distensibility (see discussion of atherosclerosis in Chapter 3). The aorta and other large vessels become stiffer with age, but they also dilate. These changes affect the cardiovascular system's efficiency in handling increased work requirements. The hearts of old rats, for example, show a reduced ability to respond to elevated arterial pressure by increasing the work of the heart (Lee et al., 1972).

Physical training in the elderly has been shown to improve their work capacity and to decrease their heart rate at rest and during work (Shock, 1977). Regular participation in exercise requiring endurance appears to be beneficial and is encouraged (Sucec, 1969). Specific information on exercise is given in Chapter 3.

Pulmonary Structure and Function

The ability of the lung to ventilate efficiently declines with age in people and animals (Liebow, 1964; Klocke, 1977; Masoro, 1979; Mauderly, 1979). The dog is the only animal on which comprehensive data have been reported (Mauderly, 1979). The lung volume of dogs, as well as people, increases in proportion to body growth until young adulthood; then the total lung volume remains relatively constant. The maximum efficiency of lung volume is reached by about one year of age in dogs and twenty years of age in people. With advancing age in both species, the capillary gas exchange becomes less efficient; maximal oxygen uptake also declines (Dill, et al., 1958; Shock, 1977). The alveoli enlarge and coalesce, with a resultant loss in elasticity and surface area. Rodents differ from dogs and people in that their lung volume increases after young adulthood. Maximum breathing capacity, as shown in Figure 6, declines more than most parameters with advancing age. Many of the changes in lung function are due to a loss of elastic recoil that occurs with advancing age, which involves the chest wall as well as the lungs (Masoro, 1979). As with cardiovascular function, physical conditioning in older individuals increases the exercise capacity and is encouraged (Tzankoff et al., 1972; see also Klocke, 1977).

Gastrointestinal Function

The capacity for digestion appears to be maintained well throughout most of life. However, adequate data are not available regarding various changes in the gastrointestinal function with age. Reports show that hydrochloric acid secretion by the stomach diminishes with advancing age, and that the secretory ability of the digestive glands decreases in elderly people (Kohn, 1971). Calcium absorption is also thought to decline with age (Bullamore et al., 1970), and the elderly may have a reduced capacity to digest protein (Masoro, 1979). Many of the problems that occur with the gastrointestinal function appear to be related to diet, the condition of the teeth, and the senses of taste and smell. It is very important for the elderly to maintain proper dental hygiene and to chew food adequately.

Taste and Smell

With advancing age, discrimination, recognition, and sensitivity in taste and smell decline (Schiffman, 1977, 1979). It seems that the bitter overwhelms the sweet in taste. One explanation is that the papillae on the back of the tongue, which sense bitterness, protrude more and are larger in old age, whereas papillae that sense saltiness and sweetness diminish remarkably in some people with age (Balogh and Lelkes, 1961). It seems sweetness and saltiness lose their intensity, as do the flavors. The decrement may be due to lack of complete cellular replacement, which in the case of taste receptors should occur every 10 days and in the nasal mucosa about every 30 days. It has been observed that the actual numbers of receptors may also decline, and the nerve pathways and the smell and taste centers in the brain degenerate. Elderly subjects, when compared with college students in a test of taste and smell of unseasoned blended foods, were found to be less able to identify the foods. The only exceptions were potatoes, tomatoes, and cabbage (Schiffman, 1977). Unfortunately, the older person may add more salt and sugar to food to compensate for taste decrement, which can have a deleterious effect on nutrition and health.

Taste can be affected by a deficiency in the diet of vitamin A, zinc, and perhaps other vitamins and minerals. Hormone levels, too, may affect taste and smell, for example, estrogen and testosterone (see Henkin, et al., 1976). Diseases such as the flu or disorders of the alimentary tract and liver, as well as hypothyroidism, can manifest themselves in a taste loss. Certain drugs can have a similar effect. Any person with a loss of taste should be instructed to maintain a balanced diet and to modify the texture of the food, for example, using chunky material rather than smooth material, and chewing better. Another great assist, as observed by Dr. Schiffman, is to add flavoring to the food. For example, strawberry and apple flavors added to food seem to increase the intake. This phenomenon is also observed in older animals such as dogs.

People who have used their sense of smell extensively throughout their life spans, such as people who deal in perfume, retain their sense of smell longer. Schiffman studied seven perfumers aged 70-78 and found less decline in both threshold and ability to discriminate odors. And five of the seven were not originally chosen as perfumers because of olfactory acuity. They very likely retained their acuity because of continual use. This is probably also true in dogs, who rely on their sense of smell and use it continuously. Although dogs may lose their hearing or even sight, I cannot recall any aged, healthy dogs that had lost their sense of smell.

Kidney Function and Acid-Base Balance

The renal system deteriorates with age. The filtration rate declines, as does the blood flow through the kidney and the kidney's ability to reabsorb glucose. There is also a decline in the functional units (glomeruli) of the kidney in rats and people with age, and this decline contributes to a decrease in urine flow (Shock and Norris, 1970; Shock, 1960, 1970, 1977; Masoro et al., 1979). The kidneys, along with the respiratory system, are involved in the very important function of maintaining the proper acidity of the cellular environment of the body within strict limits. In this respect, the kidney functions to eliminate excess acids. Studies have shown a substantial age-related difference in the body's response to dietary challenges to the acid-base balance. When 10 g of ammonium chloride was orally administered to young people, blood pH was reduced by about 0.05 units in 1½ hours. Complete recovery was observed within half a day (10 hours). However, in an 80-year-old person, this same dose of ammonium chloride produced a pH reduction three times as great, and recovery took one to three days.

In healthy individuals, however, these aging changes in the kidney are not debilitating and seem to require no special attention.

Metabolism, Temperature Regulation, and Physical Activity

Little change occurs in the basal metabolic rate with time, if one corrects for the lean body mass, which has been reported to decline with age (Bierman, 1976; Shock, 1979). The decrease in lean body mass appears to accelerate past middle age (Novak, 1972; Weg, 1978; Widdowson and Kennedy, 1962). A similar decline in lean body mass on the basis of body potassium (K^{40}) was also noted in the beagle colony at the University of California (Goldman, personal communication, 1979). In a cross-sectional study in rats of varying ages, a decline in lean body mass was also noted—but not in longitudinal studies when animals were sampled periodically during their life span. Only late in life, when the animals became ill, did their lean body mass show a decline (Lesser et al., 1973; see also Campbell et al., 1973).

Energy expenditure per unit work output, that is, work efficiency, also appears to fall as one ages. Weg (1978) suggests that older persons use more energy to perform the same amount of work.

Although heat production by functional tissue, and the maintenance of body temperature within normal limits, is little affected in the elderly, it appears that the response to high and low temperatures is less effective. The elderly seem to be able to increase heat production quite well, but their ability to conserve heat is less effective (Shock, 1977). As a result, the body temperature falls when an elderly person is exposed to cold. Of interest in this regard is a study of young and old rats, in which it was observed that after a three-minute immersion in ice water, the body temperature of the old rats fell faster and remained lower throughout the test period; their recovery rate was also slower (Thorbecke, 1975; Timiras, 1978). Thermoregulation appears to be markedly affected by age in certain mice and other animals (Finch et al., 1969; Mount, personal communication, 1979).

In my experience, keeping mice at thermal neutrality (28° C) (that is, an environmental temperature at which heat loss from the body is equal to minimum heat production) resulted in the longest-lived male mouse described in the literature up to 1960 (1,345 days) (Bustad et al., 1965). We know in animals, especially from the extensive work in pigs (Anderson, personal communication, 1979; Mount, personal communication, 1979; also his earlier publications with his associates) and other food animals, that cold and sudden changes in temperature seem to increase the incidence of disease.

I believe cold may also depress the immune system. I remember my mother telling me that during the great flu epidemic of 1918-1920 (in which she worked) one physician in her home town, as far as she could recall, never lost a case.

He had a very simple method of treatment. He insisted the patient keep very warm, avoid all chills, consume warm, nourishing food and dress warmly during recuperation. This incident has always remained with me, although when I was younger I did resist my mother's continual insistence that I dress warmly when my peers were dressing far more lightly. However, my brother and I missed very few school days because of illness; many years, we never missed a school day. The importance of warmth has remained with me for most of my life, and when I was in prison camp in the Polish corridor, I promised myself I'd never be cold again if I could help it. Yet, we still see most people in the northern climates dressing far too lightly to accommodate the cold weather conditions, especially sudden temperature changes or the colder temperatures now maintained in houses.

Setting temperatures at 18° C (65° F) or lower will have a deleterious effect on many old people who are subject to hypothermia. Clinical hypothermia is characterized by drop in deep body temperature, low peripheral blood flow, and a failure of vessels to constrict in response to cold. The defect seems to increase with age in some people (Collins et al., 1977). It can appear with the administration of certain phenothiazine drugs, for example, chlorpromazine (Jones and Meade, 1964). If the core temperature (as measured rectally) falls no lower than 90° F, human patients have a good chance of recovery. But survivors of accidental hypothermia show an impairment of their temperature regulating mechanism, which may persist for several years (MacMillan, et al., 1967). If rectal temperature falls below 80° F, death is usually the fate among the old. This also may be true with younger animals. In one of my hypothyroid sheep, the rectal temperature fell below 80° and we were unable to save its life. Between 80 and 90° F, about 70% of the human patients may be expected to survive if the exposure is not extended. Recovery is in part dependent on their alcoholic content (Weyman, 1974); we don't usually have that problem in animals. (I know of only one case, when a child during a holiday party at his home inveigled his dog into drinking the remains of the cocktails. The dog was presented to a veterinarian in a hypothermic state.)

Some elderly people, and probably some animals, are less sensitive to the sensation of cold, and therefore they may be less inclined to do what is necessary to conserve heat. It is very important they dress warmly, including long underwear and wool sweaters. The same applies to old animals; when old dogs go out in winter, especially thin dogs with sparse hair, they should wear sweaters. Maintaining laboratory animals such as rats at the comfort index of people rather than at thermal neutrality (83° F or 28° C in rats) will probably shorten their life span, especially if they are maintained beyond maturity in single housing units.

Muscular strength and stamina, along with speed of locomotion, show age-related deterioration. These changes include muscular atrophy, slowness, and a decline in motor function (Gutmann, 1977). In rats it is known that the number of muscle fibers declines with age. Very old rats show a decrease in speed of muscle contraction; the ratio of calcium transport in skeletal muscle also decreases (Gutmann, 1977; Masoro, 1976). The rate of aging may vary with the muscle group and the testing procedure. In horses, as in people, the capacity to perform light to moderate physical work does not appear to be affected appreciably by age. In some places, however, thoroughbred horses are not allowed to race after 10 or 12 years, and standard breeds are not permitted to race beyond 14 years (Reed, personal communication, 1979).

An analysis of track and field records provided data on running speed, strength, and stamina for men to age 78 and women to age 60. A gradual deterioration of speed was noted after 30 years of age. However, that deterioration was less at longer distances, suggesting that strength deteriorates faster than stamina. Beyond age 30, speed appeared to deteriorate faster for women than for men (Moore, 1975).

It is also interesting to note that the peak of muscular strength in people occurs between 20 and 30 and then

Table 3. Hormonal Changes with Advancing Age
(modified from Gregerman and Bierman, 1974)

	Hormone Concentration in Blood	Response to Stimulation	Metabolism	Action Site Sensitivity
Growth Hormone	NC*	D*		D
Thyrotropin (TSH)	NC	D		NC
Thyroxin (T4)	NC	NC	D	I*
Parathyroid hormone	D			
Adrenal androgens	D	D		
Aldosterone	D		D	
Estrogen-testosterone	D		D	

*NC = no change; D = decline; I = increase.

declines, although the rate of aging in a given muscle group varies. In an interesting study in the elderly, muscle strength at 85 years was 70% of that at 20 to 30 years. But the muscle power generated in the older men by the same muscle group cranking an ergometer, which required coordinated activity, was only slightly over 50% of the younger group (Shock and Norris, 1970). It appears that regularly performed endurance exercise increases the capacity of skeletal muscle for aerobic metabolism (Gutmann, 1977). Muscles such as the diaphragm that are continuously activated show less marked senescent changes than those less often used. As discussed in Chapter 3, exercise by the elderly may improve their health and well-being.

Hormonal Changes

The idea that aging results from failure of various endocrine glands in hormone production has been proposed for a long time. The data to support it are still being developed. Table 3 shows some of the hormonal changes that have been described (modified from Gregerman and Bierman, 1974).

Of special interest is a recent observation relative to testosterone; Finch (1978a, b) observed that testosterone declined chiefly in sick old mice, whereas in the healthy old male mice, it remained high. Testosterone levels appeared to reflect the state of health of the animal. In addition to those items included in the figure, the concentration in the blood of gonadotropins increases and triiodothyronine (T_3) concentration in the blood falls. Cortisol shows change only in its metabolism, which falls with age. Insulin shows little change except for its response to blood glucose levels, which does decline with age. It appears that the secretion of insulin is less in old subjects in response to increased blood sugar levels. It is known, of course, that glucose tolerance decreases with age, and the explanation for this seems to be decreased insulin production rather than decreased sensitivity to insulin (Masoro, 1976). Glucagon shows no change with age and the ability of the pituitary to secrete thyroid stimulating hormone (TSH), that is, thyrotropin, in response to administered thyrotropin-releasing hormone, decreases with advancing age. The remarkable complexities that characterize endocrine interrelationships and their change with age, along with our ignorance, preclude recommending any general hormone therapy for the elderly. There is, however, a possibility with increased knowledge that specific hormone therapy may be beneficial.

Nervous System

Although it is generally accepted that with old age comes a decline in the functioning of the central nervous system, many of the reported decrements in performance are due to serious diseases such as Alzheimer's disease. The often-repeated statement that we lose 100,000 neurones per day is probably a gross exaggeration (Finch, 1978b). Many age-related changes in brain function are noted, including changes in speech and voice, depression, preferential loss of short-term memory, sleep patterns, and intelligence. The last two will be given special attention.

Many of the elderly are concerned about sleep, saying they have difficulty sleeping, yet they, like many of the older animals I have worked with, do quite a bit of sleeping during the day. Data relative to sleep patterns in the elderly are conflicting. This is understandable, since only in the last 30 years have meaningful studies of sleep been conducted, and very little of the work has been performed with the elderly. With the development of brainwave recording techniques, it has been possible to record brain activity using the electroencephalograph (EEG), electrooculograph (EOG), and electromyograph (EMG). Using these techniques to study the various eye movements and associated sleep patterns, researchers discovered REM (rapid eye movement) sleep (Dement, 1972). REM sleep is referred to as "active sleep," while the non-REM is called "quiet sleep" in that it is marked by slow regular brain activity as revealed in the EEG. With REM sleep, one may observe twitches of face and fingers; there is no snoring; breathing is irregular (sometimes fast, sometimes slow). Sometimes breathing ceases for several seconds, and the eyes dart back and forth very rapidly. Blood flow and brain temperature may increase remarkably. The large muscles of the body are essentially paralyzed. When one falls asleep, one progresses through what is generally classified as four stages of non-REM sleep, with stage four being the deepest. One may then reascend through the stages of non-REM sleep and, after an hour or more, experience the first REM sleep, which may last up to 60 minutes. For someone sleeping seven to 10 hours per night, the so-called normal individual may spend one-and-one-half to two hours in REM sleep. Dreams are thought to be associated with REM sleep. Hallucinations and some dreaming occur during non-REM sleep, shortly after falling asleep.

Relative to sleep in the elderly, some researchers have stated that less sleep is required in older people. Feinberg (1969) reported that both Stage 4 and REM sleep are reduced in the elderly relative to the total sleep time. He also observed that the elderly show an increased number of awakenings and percentage of time in bed spent awake (Feinberg, 1976). Prinz and Raskind (1978) reported that so-called normal elderly, compared with young adults, demonstrated less Stage 3 and REM sleep and a loss of Stage 4.

Although some workers have suggested that neurotransmitters may have a role in the regulation of sleep, Finch (1973) stated that their role in age-related changes in sleep is highly speculative. The loss of neurones in a specialized area of the brain (locus ceruleus) during normal aging may be an important factor in the changes in the sleep patterns of the elderly (Brody, 1976).

Sleep pattern changes with age are interesting. Our 16-year-old dog (G.R.) slept more during the day than when he was younger, but not as soundly at night. That is, his deep sleep was less, as he became older, even though he had profound hearing loss. He still had periods of what appeared to be REM sleep, but they were not frequent. Although we didn't have G.R. as a pup, if he was like most dogs (my wife will probably deny that he was), REM sleep was the predominant sleep. Usually in the newborn puppy, as well as the kitten, hamster, and rat, REM sleep is thought to be the only sleep (Dement, 1972). Of interest too are data relating to bursts of growth hormone secretion during slow-wave sleep, which is reduced with age. In fact, none has been observed in older people (Roffwarg et al., 1966, Takahashi et al., 1968, Sassin et al., 1969, Carlson et al., 1972).

The difficulties with sleep that the elderly encounter may respond to some new approaches developed by Dr. Elliott Weitzman at the Sleep-Wake Disorder Center at Mountefiore Hospital in New York City, making use of a system called Chronotherapy. The Center provides a nondrug, nonpsychiatric treatment for certain sleep disorders. In certain situations, therapy begins by placing the patients on a 27-hour day, delaying their internal clock until it meshes with a more appropriate schedule. This is done in a special laboratory where the patient and the personnel do not use clocks, so there is no reference to the time of day or night. It is known as a timeless diagnostic facility (Goodwin, 1979). Most people do not have a "chronotherapist" available, but moderate exercise may help promote sleep in the elderly. At any rate, relying on drugs should not be the first choice.

That people who are old are not able to learn and perform well in intelligence tests is more fiction than fact. In a presentation entitled "Does Intelligence Decline With Age?" given at a seminar on aging research in San Francisco in November, 1977, Dr. Gisela Labouvie-Vief answered "No" with qualifications (Labouvie-Vief, 1979). One qualification was that intelligence differs with generations and also with health and vigor. Other qualifications relate to the method of testing and the testing instrument, which was originally designed for the young. It is important to understand that intelligence, in the opinion of at least some people, consists of two kinds of ability: crystallized intelligence and fluid intelligence. Crystallized intelligence is the ability to use habits of judgment based on previous experience to solve problems. This intelligence is referred to as "crystallized" because, as a result of earlier experience, it has taken on a definite form. It includes an awareness of concepts and terms and a knowledge of special fields. As one might suspect, people my age (60) did slightly better than younger people in such tests.

Older people did not do as well, however, on the fluid intelligence test, which is nonverbal, more independent of experience, and considered to be more of a test of the functioning of the nervous system. A typical question used by Dr. Labouvie-Vief was: "Some peaches are spoons. All spoons play baseball. Therefore some peaches play baseball." True or False? (This statement is true.) Many of the questions use symbols. In a study of seven generations, Dr. Labouvie-Vief noted that the decline in fluid intelligence was not evident until post retirement (after 60). And she opined that the decrement observed may have been in great part due to the manner of testing, lack of motivation, serious illness, or a general feeling of being discarded, which is common to many retired people.

She pointed out that new tests are being developed that will emphasize accuracy rather than speed and the gist of sentences and inferences rather than verbatim recall, and that these tests will emphasize tasks adults perform in everyday life. The presentation by Dr. Labouvie-Vief is consonant with the observations of many others who have recently examined comparative intelligence in the old and the young (Wilkie and Eisdorfer, 1971). I am moved at this point to repeat what I tell people when they ask how intelligent a species of animal is: I tell them it all depends on the questions one asks. This also appears to be true with the comparative intelligence of young and old people.

Relative to structural changes in the central nervous system (CNS), aging results in a loss of neurons in the CNS in animals and people, but not in all areas, and it may not occur until late in life, especially in animals (Johnson and Erner, 1972). Considerable data on brain weight has been reported, in people, but I look on this with a jaundiced eye because the extent of the brain removed is not described, and in cross-section studies I suspect that the brains of our present younger generation are larger because overall body size is greater. The brain decreases in weight from about age 35 and loses about 6 to 10 percent of its weight by old age (e.g., 70-80) (Brody and Vijayashankar, 1977). The cerebral cortex undergoes a decrease in cell numbers, but the extent of loss varies by area (Shefer, 1973). The cerebellar cortex also loses cells at a rate estimated at 25 percent by weight over an entire life span, but the loss is reported as not appreciable until the sixties in most people. In mice, no change in brain weight was observed between 10 and 30 months—and a 30-month-old mouse in some strains is very old (Finch, 1973). In some brain stem nuclei, there appears to be very little loss of cell numbers. However, in certain structures like the locus ceruleus cell loss is significant, especially in people in their seventies (Brody and Vijayashankar, 1977). Unfortunately, our data base for the nervous system is sparse. We do not know the anatomical loci of nerves that contain the various neurotransmitters, nor do we know the precise time when senescent changes occur in the many components of the nervous system, nor do we know many other items too numerous to mention (Lytle and Altar, 1979).

Diet

Dietary aspects of aging have become more important in the recent past and are actively being studied. Diet affects some of the physiological changes just discussed. Masoro and associates (1979) have spent a number of rewarding years pursuing the inadequately studied area of the effects of life-prolonging food restriction on age-related physiological changes. Their work has shown that a diet of 60 percent of a full choice intake level of feed delayed the occurrence of most age-related changes and prolonged life spans remarkably. The delayed changes included peak amount of adipose mass, decline in serum free fatty acid levels, increase in serum lipids (e.g., cholesterol), loss of muscle function and mass. Others have shown that age-related deterioration of the immune system is delayed by food restriction (Walford et al., 1974; Fernandes et al., 1976, 1978; see also Timiras, 1978; Weg, 1978) or adversely affected by excess weight (Stunkard, 1976).

The effect of food restriction goes back to the work of Osborne and associates in 1917, but it was made famous by McCay and associates (1935) at Cornell. Both these groups assigned the cause of the prolongation of the lives of rats to a retardation of growth and development early in life due to restricted caloric intake (see also Berg and Simms, 1960a, b). This has been repeatedly voiced but seldom challenged. Retarded growth and development are probably not the only reason for their results, and it may not even be the principal reason. The studies now underway by Masoro and associates will test this hypothesis—a long overdue challenge (Masoro, personal communication, 1979). On the basis of their work to date, they propose that in delaying age-related physiologic change, food restriction (using a balanced diet) retards the development of the "substratum" required for the onset of life.

Other interesting observations have been made regarding the effects of caloric restriction. Miller and Payne (1968) increased the life span of rats almost 30 percent by feeding them a high protein diet during the first four months of life and then feeding them a low protein diet thereafter. Ross and Bras (1965, 1974) have demonstrated more recently that age-related diseases in rats can be controlled by dietary manipulation and restriction (Masoro, personal communication, 1979; see also Cohen, 1979). If applied late in life, however, such restriction may in fact shorten the life span. No one really knows what is happening in these rats and whether, in fact, the findings have anything to say about the situation in human beings, nonhuman primates, or pigs. In all probability they do, and such work is important to pursue (Hollander, 1978). It is noteworthy that rats, given free choice, will choose a diet that is probably most deleterious to them, and in that regard they are very much like people (see Ross and Bras, 1974; Ross, 1959, 1976, 1978). In the not-too-distant future, the "experiment" on dietary reduction will involve many people and probably fewer rats, whether we like it or not. With an increasing population and a diminished plane of nutrition, much of the world's population will be experimental subjects throughout their lifetime. It is up to those who remain to make it as useful an experiment as possible, so that those people who are on a damagingly low plane of nutrition, and whose diet is unbalanced, may have the best quality of life possible under adverse circumstance. It appears, however, that little can be gained by severe dietary restriction of the elderly except in special cases such as severe hypertension, diabetes, or severe hyperlipidemia.

Theories

Age-related changes in structural and physiological functions have served as a basis for the development of a number of hypotheses and theories about aging. The prevailing theories to explain physiological aging that I reviewed twenty years ago were:

- The accumulation of extracellular and intracellular injurious materials in the form of bacterial toxins, hydrolytic enzymes such as phosphatases and esterases, and free radicals (short-lived reactive chemical compounds in the body), all leading to altered metabolic activity (Metchnikoff, 1907; Bourne, 1956; Harman, 1956, 1960; see also Gordon, 1974)

- Physiochemical changes in colloids, with cellular and intercellular accumulation of structural obstacles to metabolism, filtration, transport, and diffusion, all leading to a decline in metabolic activity because of a diminishing ability of the circulatory system to meet the demands of the cell (Childs, 1915; Dhar, 1926, 1930; Brody, 1945; Lansing, 1952)
- Exhaustion of a fixed reserve in the organism, as revealed by data suggesting equivalent numbers of calories per unit weight consumed per lifetime in several mammals, or depletion of specific cell constituents in the postmitotic cell —for example, certain enzyme molecules that exhibit finite lives in terms of turnover
- Gene mutation or chromosome damage in the somatic cell (or germ cell) leading to a deteriorating cell population, a consequence of a faulty copying mechanism (Muller, 1951; see also Comfort, 1956, for Dr. Surway's proposal, and see Comfort, 1964, 1979)
- Disturbance in stable state of equilibrium in the body we call homeostasis, which is a result of changes in response-time of target organs in complex feedback systems.

These five general hypotheses are still being discussed. Some have been modified and extended and new ones have appeared. Fortunately, some very early theories have fallen by the wayside. Indeed, this was the fate of one of the most publicized of the early theories proposed by Brown-Sequard in 1889. He believed that aging of the gonads was the key factor in aging, and claimed that testicular extracts had a rejuvenating action (Andres and Tobin, 1977). If this were true, castrated animals and people should have abnormal life spans; yet I know of no evidence to support this premise. Perhaps T. H. Huxley (1888) was right when he said that a theory is a species of thinking, and its right to exist is coextensive with its power to resist extinction by its rivals. In more recent times, Nathan Shock (1974), the grand old man of modern gerontology, said that one of the problems with that discipline was that there are too many hypotheses and too few data to test them.

It is very difficult to give a balanced view of the current aging theories; many fine reviews have appeared. (See Rockstein et al., 1974; Finch and Hayflick, 1977; Weg, 1978; Strehler, 1977; Cutler, 1978; Behnke et al., 1978; Timiras, 1978; Comfort, 1979.) I will first address some of the extensions of the theories I reviewed 20 years ago, beginning with inhibitory and toxic substances produced in the body. This is followed by a longer presentation on the exciting developments that have occurred in the area of cellular aging, showing cultures of most tissues are not ageless but "run out of program." This discussion reflects the very productive effort in cellular, biochemical, and molecular aspects of aging in the recent past (Brash and Hart, 1978). For sake of completeness, I will discuss the wear-and-tear hypothesis in view of its relationship to the possible effects of free choice of activity. The discussion on the immune system, autoimmunity, and viruses (including slow viruses) reflect the prodigious effort that many workers in these fields have made during the last two decades. The review of aging theories ends with a summary of the recent thinking regarding aging clocks and the neuroendocrine control of the aging process.

Some of the earliest theories concerned inhibitory or toxic substances produced in the body that are deleterious to maintaining a "steady state." Many agents have been suggested, including deuterium, calcium, bacterially produced toxins in the intestines—but these are no longer considered important. Free radicals have already been mentioned. The significance of cross-linking products and age pigments in the aging process is still being discussed. The cross-linking of collagen and other components, such as polyunsaturates, is observed and still promoted (Strehler, 1977; Bjorksen, 1968, 1974). It has been suggested that age-related changes are most applicable in noncellular parts of the body, that is, intercellular spaces, where they can deleteriously affect the flexibility and efficiency of muscles, including the heart, the movement of substances from blood to cells, and the oxygenation of tissue (Weg, 1978).

As Strehler (1977) says in his inimitable style, cross-linking of certain substances makes them very useful for the paint and varnish industry, but "the gradual accumulation of a layer of varnish on certain biological structures is an unpleasant prospect." The data are insufficient to specify cause and effect but we cannot deny that cross-linking does occur with advancing age and also that aging pigments accumulate. Lipofuscin, an aging pigment, is higher in the hearts of Japanese who consume more unsaturated fats than Westerners, which may or may not be significant (Strehler, 1977).

In the 1950s, when I was writing my thesis, it seemed that everyone believed most cells in culture were immortal. Every "well-read" person referred to the chicken heart fibroblasts Alexis Carrel (1935) had kept in culture for many decades. It wasn't until Hayflick's (1965) work on human fibroblasts that Carrel's "immortal" cells were declared mortal. It seems that in the technique Carrel used, when embryo extract was periodically added to his culture media, small numbers of embryonic cells also were added. Hayflick and associates showed that human fibroblasts in culture would go through 50 to 60 doublings, manifesting in late stages a progressive exhaustion of growth potential. When Hay and Strehler (1967) repeated Carrel's work on chicken fibroblasts, he found the number of doublings was only about 20 (15-35). We now know, from techniques used by Hayflick and others (Hayflick, 1980), that normal cells from people and other mammals have a limited capacity to divide, and it is a reflection of the life of the particular species or the age of the animal from which the tissue is obtained.

The evidence available suggests a direct relationship between the life span of the species and the capacity of its cells to divide in culture. The exceptions are cancer cells, which may multiply indefinitely, and the germ cells, the sperm and egg and their precursors. It has been suggested these cells may escape senescence by the sharing and reshuffling of genetic material (e.g., by viruses, chemicals, or by fusion of sperm and egg).

In reflecting on the finiteness of normal cells in culture, Hayflick (1975) suggested that animals age not so much because cell populations cease dividing in the body but more probably because metabolic changes that develop before the cessation of doubling and death are more critical and lead to disturbed structure and function. The work of Hayflick and others suggests that the cells from most tissues are programmed genetically with an inborn clock that dictates a cell's ability to replicate (or multiply). A number of people have shown that, by replacing the nucleus in an old cell with a young nucleus or by putting an old nucleus in a young cell, the clock that determines the ability of the cell to continue to divide is controlled by the nucleus.

It has long been suggested that one's heredity is important in determining length of life. When people ask me how long they could expect to live, I give them the same answer that Sir John Hammond gave me when I asked him this question. He said, "I'll answer you in the words that Pearl gave me early in this century: 'If you want a long life span, pick a mother and grandparents with a long life span.' " (Pearl, 1928)

Studies comparing 1,600 pairs of twins, identical (monozygotic) twins with fraternal (dizygotic) ones, revealed that heredity is a factor (Kallmann and Sander, 1949). The average difference in the age of death for identical twins was less than that of fraternal twins (Jarvik, et al., 1960).

Apparently, contradictory data have appeared in the follow-up studies of some of the descendants of Pearl's nonagenarians. Only a slight correlation was found between age of death of grandparents and that of their descendants. This finding, however, probably can be explained by the great improvement in modern medicine and nutrition that has extended the life spans of descendants of both short-lived and long-lived people (Moment, 1978). Those possibly destined for a short life benefited from modern medicine and lived longer than their parents.

The rate of living—or metabolic rate—theory was proposed by Rubner in 1908. The theory has been espoused by many people, including Pearl, and is still being discussed. Since this theory assumes an organism "wears out," it is sometimes called the "wear-and-tear" theory. The theory maintains that with increased metabolism and higher temperatures, the calories burn sooner and, therefore, the life span decreases. Rubner suggested that several mammals seem to consume about the same number of calories per kilogram of body weight (200,000 kcals/kg) during their life span, regardless of size. Generally, animals also seem to have about the same number of heartbeats during their life span—whether mouse or elephant (Asimov, 1965; Moment, 1978). It is intriguing that at the end of a life span the very rapidly beating heart of a 3½-year-old mouse will have contracted as many times (roughly about 1×10^9) as the slowly beating heart of an elephant my age. The basal metabolic rate and temperature of individual animals seems to be related to life span. People, though, are an exception to these generalities. For example, in the past 60 years I have probably consumed about 600,000 kilocalories per kilogram of body weight, and my heart has beaten about three times more often than that of a 70-year-old elephant.

At Johns Hopkins University it was observed that the life of fruit flies could be doubled or cut in half by either raising or lowering the temperature in which they live (Moment, 1978). Men, who have a high metabolic rate, are outlived by women. Work at the University of Southern California by Strehler (1977) has shown that mice with lower body temperatures usually live much longer.

Rubner's concept probably contributed to the wear-and-tear theory, and many people readily accepted it considering that if a fuel burns very fast, it is used up sooner. However, this concept is in conflict with the idea that activity is good, and that people who are active are healthier and presumably longer lived than those who are very sedentary. Neither of these notions had any confirmation within a species until Sacher and Duffy (1979) performed an interesting study at Argonne National Laboratory.

Sacher took five inbred strains of mice and mated them. He obtained 25 different crosses; the offspring of these crosses were used in the experiment. He measured metabolic rates for samples of each genotype and also kept samples of each genotype for life span. He ended up with a set of metabolic rates and a set of life span data. Findings showed that animals with the highest metabolic rate had the shortest life spans, and those with the lowest had the longest life spans. These observations tended to confirm Rubner and to satisfy the intuitive understanding that when something ran fast it reached the endpoint sooner.

But it contradicted the other idea that being active was inherently good, because it meant that any amount of activity would require extra metabolic activity and shorten life. So he reexamined all of his data and in particular the 24-hour cycle of activity and of rest for each different genotype. Each genotype might show a difference in resting metabolic rate, but it could also differ independently on the amplitude of its daily cycle of activity. Therefore, he took a measure expressed as the ratio of the average metabolism to the resting metabolism. This ratio expressed the relative magnitudes of the two rates, which was that fraction of the animal's total metabolism that it was able to put into its daily cycle of activity. The cycle of activity above the minimum resting value is the energy available to the animal for meeting its needs, such as moving, grooming, eating, mating, or responding to environmental challenge. Sacher called this ratio the Activity Index, and plotted life span against it for the same genotypes. It turned out that the animals with a high Activity Index were longer lived than those with a lower Index. This seemed to bear out the other intuitive idea that he, I, and others shared, that activity per se is good and maintains health and supports life.

Actually, the two contradictory intuitions we have about metabolism and life span may both be true. In other words, they are different aspects of the way in which life depends upon metabolism. On the one hand, metabolism achieves all the things involved in protecting the organism against fluctuations, infections, and environmental attacks, while giving it stability and extending its life, but on the other, the activity wears out the organism. Living, at least for higher organisms, seems to involve finding a balance and getting the most out of metabolic activity in spite of the inevitable, inescapable attrition that comes from activity itself. What we need to do when talking about how individuals achieve a longer life is to find an optimum Activity Index. The data suggest that an optimum amount exists for any activity. We certainly can not conclude that if an activity is good, then ten times as much is better. That attitude is causing great problems today when it is applied to exercise, vitamins, and dietary fads. I believe that moderate activity is better than none, but I also feel that freely chosen, healthful, pleasurable activity is more beneficial than uninvited, coerced activity. Freedom, celebration, fun, play, and laughter are healthful for man and beast. Definitive work should address this issue.

Data from some of Kavanau's work (1963) suggest that animals prefer options and appear more prone to exercise if the exercise wheel goes in either direction. Kavanau holds the view that almost all operant testing approaches to measure an animal's ability are inadequate because they do not give the animal choices, whereas animals usually have choices in more natural situations. When Kavanau set up a running wheel so that the animal could use it at any time or in any direction, he obtained totally different behavior patterns than when the wheel was set up to go only in one direction or only at prescribed times. The running of these same animals was governed by the phases of the moon. Kavanau used an artificial moon and found that animals would run the wheel at certain times and in certain directions; if the wheel were locked so that the animals could run in only one direction, they did not run at all. If the wheel were opened so that they could run in either direction, they would run indefinitely.

We need to conduct an experiment that combines an "activity" environment with choices and test the effect on life span compared with standard handling methods, which may be extremely anxiety producing. We should also combine activity with restricted or free choice situations, such as Masoro (personal communication, 1979) and his associates are doing. The relevance of these animal data to people is tenuous at this state of knowledge. Certainly the Activity Index, that is, the ratio of the average metabolic rate to the resting rate of Sacher's mice, falls with advancing age, as it does with people. I interpret the data to mean that we need as many options for activity as possible to provide interest and diversity, while using as many muscles, joints, and functions (both mental and physical) as possible. Also, we need to adjust our activity to a level appropriate for our age.

One theory of aging relates the decline in the immune function and the increase in autoantibodies to advancing age. The immune system, which is programmed to recognize and attack foreign material, fails to recognize "self" and attacks it as foreign, that is, self-recognition is lost. Proponents believe that this age change in the immune system is primarily responsible for the failure of important cell functions that culminates in death (Walford, 1969). With the failure of the immune system, an individual is more vulnerable to disease. Although our knowledge is incomplete, we think the immune response is mediated principally by two classes of white blood cells, called T-cells and B-cells (lymphocytes). Both types of cell develop after birth, in most mammals, from a stem cell in the bone marrow. T-cells mature in the thymus, and B-cells somewhere else, probably in the bone marrow and lymphoid tissue. B-cells in the chicken, for instance, mature in the bursa of Fabricius (Perryman, 1979). These cells are involved in what is referred to as the *cell-mediated immune response* to a foreign material, contrasted to a *humoral immune response,* which is characterized by synthesis and release of antibodies. B-cells are most involved in antibody production. Adler (1975) has provided evidence that the activity of T-cells decreases with age faster than similar activity of B-cells. Although an older individual may form adequate antibodies in response to a vaccine, there appears to be an age-related failure to retain antibody levels (Blankwater, 1978; see McKinodan, 1978; Kumar, 1979).

It is generally assumed that the changes in cellular immune function are more prominent than changes in the humoral immune function, where the change appears to be more qualitative than quantitative. In work by Kruisbeek (1978), the thymus-dependent immune function (i.e., cellular immune function) was depressed in aging rats and in rats with tumors. But the cause for depression was different in the two models. In the old rats, the number of active T-cells declined, whereas in tumor-bearing animals the ability of T-cells to multiply and to function properly was impaired. It appears that in aged animals the environment of the thymus, whatever remains of it, is not conducive to proper maturation of the T-cells, and the bone marrow apparently changes so that the early form of the B-cells may be affected (Kruisbeek, 1978).

We have not yet reached the stage in research where we can recommend a thymus-derived "hormone" or other compound to delay, reverse, or prevent immunosenescence or to reverse the immunosuppression seen in some cancers. But I believe sufficient evidence already exists that we can be somewhat optimistic that we may find a means for delaying the onset of, or minimizing the severity of, certain diseases of the elderly by manipulating the immune system, especially cell-mediated immunity. I do not, however, wish to underestimate the complexity of the immune system. Nothing exemplifies this complexity better than the situation with viruses, including slow viruses.

It has been proposed that repeated viral infections of various types throughout life cause an individual to develop a "library" of viral genetic information that contributes to the decline in physiological function with age. With a decline in the activity of cell-mediated immunity, virally infected tissue (under the surveillance of ailing lymphocytes) is no longer recognized as self but as foreign tissue and is attacked by antiviral or antitissue antibodies, thus explaining the cause of increased autoantibodies in the elderly (Adler, 1974). But diseased tissue may not be rejected, which may set the stage in some way for tumor production and other aging phenomena (Adler, 1974).

In the fifties, Sigurdsson (1954) described a group of animal diseases in which, after initiation of the viral infection, a long latent period that may extend into years was followed by clinical signs of illness, usually ending in severe disease or death. That is how the slow virus story began. Interest in slow and latent viruses has proliferated in the recent past; in fact, Gajdusek shared the Nobel prize recently for his work on slow viruses. Although there is no direct evidence that these viruses are involved in any progressive, degenerative changes associated with senescence, this has been proposed (Gajdusek, 1974; Meek, 1977). It is known that many viruses, some of them common, may persist in latent or defective form after an acute illness, such as measles, and then decades later cause lesions. These may develop either from the direct action of the virus on cells, or from continual deposition of viral immune complexes at various sites in the vascular system. It is proposed that these persistent infections may be responsible for the degenerative changes one sees in aging, such as those involved in kuru and Creutzfeldt-Jakob disease, scrapie in sheep (Hadlow, 1959), and others. Although slow viruses do not always destroy cells, they impair their functioning. An infection by slow viruses shows little evidence of inflammatory response to suggest that they are infectious. These diseases are called spongiform virus encephalopathies. They evoke a slow loss of neurons and other changes of the supporting structures of the central nervous system that resemble the pathologic changes seen in the aging nervous system. This is certainly an interesting proposal and an area for investigation.

Oldstone and Dixon (1974) also feel viruses are able to persist, especially in neurons and lymphocytes, and suppress their unique function for long periods of time and contribute to what we see as aging.

Considerable research has been done recently on the subject of aging clocks. One of the more articulate spokesmen, Everitt (1973), states that most hormones accelerate the aging process in their target organs in one way or another. This stimulation increases the functional load on these organs and increases the wear and tear on them. He, therefore, proposed an aging hormone as one that would increase physiological aging or the pathology associated with it. He went on to state that although there is little evidence for the existence of a general aging hormone, a number of organ-aging hormones appear to be regulated by the hypothalamic-pituitary-peripheral endocrine system. He further stated that the environmental factors that accelerate and shorten life do so by increasing the secretion of these various aging hormones. Denckla (1975, 1977) also promoted the idea of a regulatory mechanism more associated with death than with aging. Applying several lines of reasoning, he suggested that death, as opposed to aging, is a regulated function in mammals and that the hypothalamic-pituitary axis may well be the site for regulation of the time that death occurs. Most proposals regarding the aging clock state that its location is in the hypothalamus region at the base of the brain. In support of this, the advocates point out that the control of growth, and also the development and activities of the gonads, the thyroid and many other glands, are located in the hypothalamic area.

Caleb Finch, at the University of Southern California, has actively pursued research in this area and has made some very interesting observations (Finch, 1969, 1975, 1976, 1977, 1978a, b). Finch et al. (1969, 1978) believe that the brain controls, or at least influences, most cell and organ functions via nerves and/or hormones. The brain and the pituitary are important components of the control system. Finch and others have proposed that some aging changes in the brain may cause hormonal shifts (Finch and Hayflick, 1977; Clemens et al., 1978; Finch, 1979). Catecholamines (like adrenalin) are important relative to controlling cycles, e.g., the reproductive cycle. They are thought to act as neurotransmitters in many parts of the nervous system. Levodopa, used to treat Parkinson's disease, is converted to catecholamines in the brain. Finch and others have shown that aging reduces brain catecholamine metabolism in the hypothalamus and other parts of the brain (like the basal ganglia, which is affected in Parkinson's disease, with more than 80% depletion of dopamine). Recently it has been shown that dopamine depletion occurs in both mice and people, and the extent of depletion is remarkably proportionate to the life span. It is not, however, as severe as that seen in Parkinson's. Cotzias, who introduced levodopa treatment of Parkinson's disease, found using high dosages of this drug increased the life span and reduced the incidence of tumors in one type of laboratory mice (Cotzias et al., 1977).

Finch and others remind us that there is really no steady state for our body functions; they are in a dynamic state and continue to change with time. Since the hypothalamus (to which the pituitary gland is attached) controls so many glands, its influence on aging and its central control must be considered seriously. The complex relationship between brain, hormones, and tissues explains the dynamic state of metabolism, with one change causing a cascade of events that may explain many of the aging phenomena (Finch, 1979).

The nature of the mechanism for control has been suggested as a gradual elevation of the threshold of sensitivity of the hypothalamic area to normal feedback from the endocrine glands. It can be likened to a furnace that becomes less and less responsive to a thermostat. As a result, it pours out too much heat before it turns off, or the room has to get too cold before the furnace turns on and sends out heat. The suggested sites are in the biochemical properties of cell membranes, which may be involved in circadian rhythms in both plants and animals. The "clock" may well be governed to an extent by the amount of protective redundancy, i.e., excess, of genetic information or the effectiveness of the DNA repair mechanism, both of which are under genetic control.

At this incomplete stage of our knowledge, as a physiologist I am attracted by the proposal that aging is a failure in the neuroendocrine control mechanisms. In animals and people, the deteriorations one observes are greatest in performance tests that require the coordinated activities of a number of systems rather than just a single one. A good deal of evidence suggests that the neurotransmitters go out of "balance" (see Timiras and Bignami, 1976; Timiras, 1978; Finch, 1978, 1979, and personal communication). Some neurotransmitters show decrements, whereas others do not. Timiras (1978) proposed that the higher brain centers are the "pacemakers" that regulate the biological clock that controls not only growth and development, but aging and death. She thinks that, with aging, the activity of the brain cortex, the hypothalamus, the pituitary, and other endocrine glands (along with agents and organs that regulate them) is impaired. Any slowing down would then affect the neurotransmitters, which would ultimately depress muscle and joint function, cardiovascular function, the immune mechanism, and many secretions and other functions and systems. The result would be decrement in our adaptive ability and our general well-being. The proposals relative to neuroendocrine aspects of aging are interesting because many aspects are testable. In fact, many scientists are productively pursuing varied aspects of neuroendocrine control.

Prospects

Many theories of aging continue to compete for prominence. Actually, most theories have elements of truth that are now being evaluated. Many people fondly hope that, with genetic manipulation or other means, human life may be extended indefinitely. I do not cherish this hope nor wish to live here indefinitely. A Greek myth captured the agony of continuing to age but never dying: The goddess Eos persuaded Zeus to grant the man Tithonus immortality but forgot to ask for eternal youth. He grew gray and feeble and finally was locked away where Eos could not hear his babbling.

It is of interest to me that for a long time, three score and ten has described the length of life for most people. We enjoy reading about exceptions, but must remember they are exceptions. Changes one sees with time are normal deteriorations of function that are inevitable and can be tolerable. As Jefferson said, "There is a fullness of time when men should go and not occupy too long the ground to which others have a right to advance." During my life and yours, we will not see a replacement therapy regimen that will modify three score and ten appreciably, although there are indications that if one limits dietary intake in early and middle years and is moderate, a substantial lengthening of the effective life span may be possible (Masoro, personal communication, 1979).

Some suggestions for prolonging life were comprehensively discussed by Sacher (1977); ethical aspects of this have been discussed more recently (Veatch, 1979). Of special interest, in addition to the effectiveness of dietary restriction, is that of body and environmental temperature. A mean body temperature just one degree above normal (39° C) shortened the life span of rats. Body temperatures below 39° C were not correlated with life span (Kibler and Johnson, 1966; Carlson et al., 1957). It appears important to maintain individuals near their comfort index or at an environmental temperature not requiring increased metabolism for cooling or heating by the individual, that is, at thermal neutrality. The other item of recurring interest is the possible beneficial effects of procaine, which has been reported to help old people (Aslan, 1965). In rats, it was found that frequent administration improved the psychophysiological performance and reduced disease incidence and mortality rate. Its general application to people is still debated.

All about us we see involutional degeneration and death in normal development. These deteriorations and deaths are predictable at specific times in the life span of the mammals that I know. Some of the examples of these are deciduous teeth that are replaced, the baby fat of childhood, the placenta during gestation, the changes in the ovary and uterus of females, the thymus gland of the young. The late Hardin Jones recognized these changes that "appear to occur characteristically at an age as though they may be the endpoints of other processes" as he developed an argument for a theory of aging that was based, not on programmed changes, but on accumulated disease experience. He proposed that each disease experience was an "increment of damage" that contributed to the physiological progression of aging, with each increment becoming more intense and leaving its mark (Jones, 1956). When I discussed this proposal at some length with Hardin Jones in 1958, he elaborated and explained it further. He drew on the blackboard a series of curves, which I have modified and redrawn for illustrative purposes (Figure 6). As explained earlier in this chapter, if we express mortality or disease incidence as a function of age (the Gompertz plot), we obtain a relatively straight line for much of an animal's or person's life, which makes comparison easier.

With each increment of damage in Figure 6, an individual moves to a new line with a reduced life expectancy. The bottom heavy line is the curve for an individual with the maximum life expectancy, for example, a woman living in rural Sweden, who is married and has children. A cigarette smoker could expect to die 5-10 or more years sooner than the Swedish woman, depending in part on the intensity of the habit. In the same way, city residence, singleness, alcohol abuse, or obesity would affect an individual's position on the curve. For illustrative purposes, an overweight bachelor living in Brooklyn who smoked two packs a day could decrease his life expectancy by about 35 years. Unfortunately, almost everything that happens to us shifts us to a curve denoting an earlier departure from life—that is the bad news! The

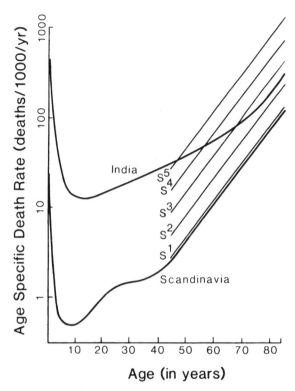

Figure 6. Age-specific mortality for various subpopulations exposed to disease experiences or other increments of damage owing to life-style or environmental hazards. Deleterious experiences, e.g., smoking or overeating, result in an upward shift to a new curve and a predictably shorter life span.

good news is that with the elimination of these "increments of damage," for example, smoking, drinking, alcohol, overeating, many of us could assume a more favorable curve for a longer, healthier life span.

I take heart from the knowledge that many people stay keen of mind and body and experience relatively good health until very late in life. They are able to make great contributions into their seventies, eighties, and nineties (Figures 7-10).

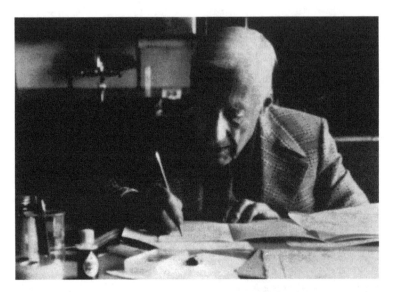

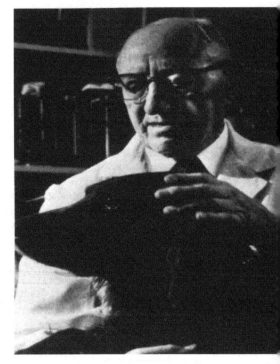

Figure 7. Joel Hildebrand, an
outstanding teacher and
scientist at the University of
California at the age of 97.

Figure 8. Edward Boyden,
a prolific scientist until
age 89, and his constant
companion Tara.

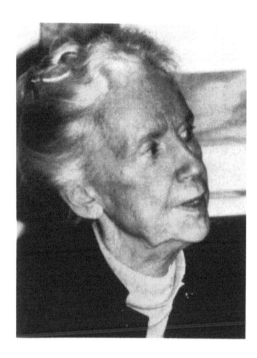

Figure 9. Maggie Kuhn, cofounder of the Gray Panthers.

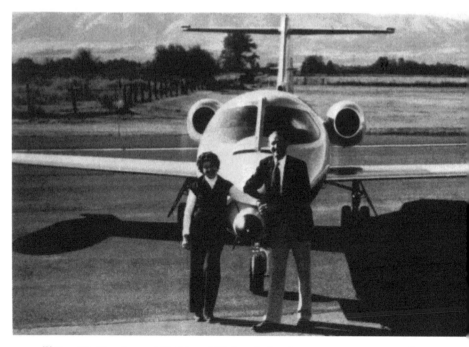

Figure 10. Maurice and Kathleen Hitchcock, lumber company owners, pilots, and enthusiastic racehorse owners in Washington state.

Brain is like a muscle—if you do not use it, you lose it. This is the philosophy of five remarkable people—the famous chemist, Dr. Joe Hildebrand, who is still teaching and publishing at the University of California at the age of 97 (Figure 7); the great anatomist, Edward Boyden, an active scientist until 89 (Figure 8); Maggie Kuhn, the delightful cofounder of the Gray Panthers, who has a lecture schedule that would challenge anyone half her age (Figure 9); and Maurice and Kathleen Hitchcock, enthusiastic racehorse owners, pilots, and lumber company owners (Figure 10). All five of them share three important characteristics: They keep busy, keep interested, and do not lose their sense of humor. Maurice said of his wife Kathleen, "She's a slow learner! She didn't obtain instrument rating on our Lear jet until she was 69."

These people should encourage us to strive for a longer, healthier, more useful, and rewarding life. By applying much of what we already know, we can accomplish this for a significant number of people. Much of our success relates to how we treat one another, but nutrition and life style are also basic. Some of our knowledge can be usefully applied to the elderly now, and much of it can be used by the elderly to help educate their grandchildren so that they may have better prospects than their grandparents for a healthy life. The primary motive in this book is to enable such applications.

CHAPTER 3

ANIMAL CONTRIBUTIONS TO GERIATRIC MEDICINE

This subject of man's body is of all other things in nature most susceptible of remedy; but then that remedy is most susceptible of error. For the same subtlety of the subject doth cause large positivity and easy failing; and therefore the inquiry ought to be the more exact.

Sir Francis Bacon

Health professionals owe an enormous debt to animals, for studies of various species have provided essential understanding of major human health problems. As a veterinarian, I have spent much of my scientific career observing animals, and hope to turn my observations and those of my colleagues into helpful suggestions for the benefit of the elderly and all those who contribute to their health and well-being. As background to my discussion of heart disease and cancer research, I would like to begin with an elementary prerequisite: An appreciation of the uniqueness of each living organism (person or animal) is essential to understanding and caring for that organism. It is critical that every member of the health delivery team realize the elderly are far more diverse than any other age group. As Dr. Robert Butler, Director of the National Institute of Aging, said recently, "We become more complicated as we grow older" (Butler, 1975, and personal communication, 1979).

Whether of man or beast, individuality is too often unrecognized. We have no difficulty in accepting that people are

55

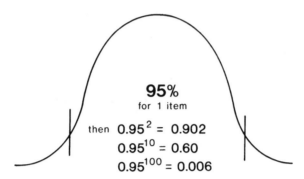

Figure 11. A normal bell-shaped distribution curve encompasses 95% of normal individuals for two variables, 60% for 10 variables, and .6% for 100 variables.

tall, short, fat, and thin, or that no two people look exactly alike. Yet we classify most beings as "average" in spite of all their differences, and so make judgments and prescribe therapy. Sir William Osler, quoting Parry of Bath, stated it well: "It is more important to know what sort of patient has a disease than to know what sort of a disease a patient has."

The subject of variability among people has been given short shrift (Williams, 1956). A normal, bell-shaped distribution curve (with two standard deviations of the mean) typically encompasses 95% of the people and labels them "normal," assuming only 5% of the population are abnormal. But a host of measurable attributes dispute this classification. We must realize that in a sample of 1,000 people, even if 950 of the population is "normal" for one variable, only 900 will be normal for two measureable variables, 600 for 10. About six "normal" or "average" people occur per 1,000 when we consider 100 variables (Williams, 1956) (Figure 11).

The only reasonable conclusion we can draw is that everyone is unique; everyone is handicapped, "abnormal," or unusual. Mothers are right: "No one's baby is like mine." (Although when these same babies become teenagers, many parents are quite certain the babies must have been switched in the hospital at birth, and they ended up with the wrong one.) In Medawar's interesting book (1957) on the uniqueness of the individual, he related an event in which monozygotic (identical) twins had been "muddled up" in the hospital. The mistake was not discovered until the boys were 6 years old and resemblance revealed the real twin brother. The disputed parentage was determined by utilizing small skin grafts on the three children involved. In relating this, Dr. Medawar highlighted the uniqueness of each individual, as determined by the immune system.

Anatomical, physiological, and biochemical variability in the same species was impressed upon me when I joined General Electric Company's Hanford Laboratories in 1949. My first project was to perform a lifelong study in sheep to determine the biological effects of radioiodine when administered over their lifetimes. In performing radioiodine uptakes in the thyroid, I found that for a given group of 12 sheep of the same age (purebred Suffolks obtained from one producer), the iodine uptakes varied by up to a factor of 10. The weight of thyroids also varied greatly, as did weights of some other organs.

One of the few studies on anatomical variations was performed in rabbits over 50 years ago. Brown and co-workers (1926) collected data on organ weights in 645 normal male adult rabbits from stock used for experimental purposes. The range of organ weights was remarkable (Table 4).

Ranges of up to 10 were relatively commonplace, with the spleen showing a ratio from the maximum to minimum weight of 80. In view of these and other observations in a relatively select group of purebred animals (some of them even inbred), one can expect that in human beings the variation may be far greater and, therefore, of even more consequence. These anatomical variations extend to form, size, and shape of a structure, the connections of certain ducts, and the composition and requirements.

Soon after joining Hanford Laboratories, I met Roger

Table 4. Relative Organ Weights of Rabbits (modified
from Brown, et al., 1926)

Organ	Ratio of Minimum to Maximum Weights
Spleen	80
Thyroid	25
Parathyroid	22
Lymph notes, deep cervical	15
Lymph nodes, axillary	13
Thymus	13
Pineal	12
Testicle	10
Mesenteric lymph nodes	10
Adrenals	7
Pituitary, kidneys, and liver	5
Brain	2.5
Heart	2

Williams from the University of Texas, who spoke on individuality from the perspective of a nutritionist and biochemist.
He speculated that variation in individual nutritional needs
might offer the solution to many baffling health problems.
Although variability was one of the commonly observed phenomena in all studies, no one had really quantitated it. He
began collecting information and published a book entitled
Biochemical Individuality. In the book's preface, Alan Gregg
stated that students of human biology, especially in clinical
work, need to be "chary of assuming uniformly sufficient
single causation or cause for events." He reminded us we
need to remember not merely the environment but also that
every organism brings its own environment from the past, its
heredity. Relative to heredity, one must be mindful of almost
infinite interplay of genetic factors. Hereditary factors are
certainly manifest in body structure as well as disease susceptibility.

The meaning of "average" or "mean" has little significance.
Hoffer (1977) stated, in this regard, that two main types of
error exist, error of the means and error of the extremes. The
first is perpetuated by well-meaning people who firmly ad-
here to the mean requirement laid down in the tables listing

nutritional requirements and advise everyone to do likewise. However, they miss the extremes. The second error occurs when a person finds what is best for him or her and immediately concludes it must be the best for everyone. Thus, someone may recommend "healthy" food items that are a boon to one person but that may unfortunately cause problems for others. We have a long way to go in objectively seeking optimum nutrition for each individual.

In the field of animal nutrition, especially for chickens, dogs, cats, pigs, and dairy cows, we provide good nutrition. Animal diets usually contain high-quality protein and sufficient vitamins and minerals to promote near optimum growth, health, and production. We have not reached these same goals with people. We must recognize that every person, young or old, although appearing "normal" may have an abnormality that bears on his or her nutritional requirement as well as susceptibility to disease and ability to "cope."

With the idea of individual variability firmly in mind, we can now consider the greatest problems of the elderly to which animals have contributed significantly to our understanding and management. The diseases to be discussed are those which the elderly regard as important to them, namely, coronary heart disease, cancer, osteoporosis, periodontal disease, and mental disorders. Few people would disagree that these are among the most troubling and costly for the elderly.

We must prepare our students well in geriatric medicine, for those training now will be in the prime of their professional career in twenty years when one half their patients will be over 65 years of age, and one-half the federal health bill will be spent on this age group. Since many regard the greatest challenge in the western world to be coronary heart disease, and since studies of animals have helped us understand this disease, it will be reviewed first.

Coronary Heart Disease – Atherosclerosis

A discussion of coronary heart disease (CHD) necessarily concentrates on atherosclerosis, which is involved in almost all coronary heart disease. Atherosclerosis is a disorder

Table 5. Chain of Events in Atherosclerosis

1. Endothelial injury	Chemical (e.g., homocystine) Mechanical (shear forces) Immunologic Chronic lipidemia

2. Endothelial loss

3. Platelet adherence, aggregation and release of constituents

4. Platelet constituent(s) stimulate(s) smooth muscle proliferation

5. Connective tissue formation

6. Calcification of lesion(s)

7. Thrombosis and infarction

See Ross and Glomset, 1973; 1976; Ross and Harker, 1976; Kottke and Subbiah, 1978.

characterized by elevated plaques and by thickenings called atheromas within the blood vessels (Table 5). These atheromas cause mischief by undergoing calcification, internal hemorrhages, ulceration, and sometimes superimposed thrombosis. This chain of events is seldom observed in animals in the so-called natural state.

Atherosclerosis, along with hypertension, dominates human morbidity and mortality statistics in North America and much of Western Europe. Atherosclerosis is the number one killer of the elderly. Studies of animals in their "natural" state suggest that their low incidence of atherosclerosis may be attributed to life style, diet, and relatively short lifespan. Modification of animals' natural diet and other manipulations induce atherosclerosis in most species.

The complexities of atherosclerosis were indelibly im-

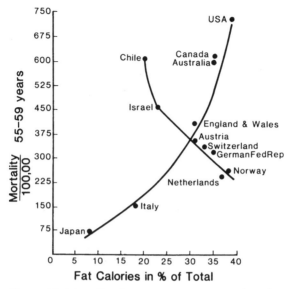

Figure 12. Mortality from heart disease as a function of fat consumption (adapted from Keys, 1953 and Gudbrandsen, 1961).

pressed on me when I attended the University of Washington School of Medicine in the late fifties as a postdoctoral fellow. An associate, Cato Ohrn Gudbrandsen (in Loren Carlson's laboratory), became interested in diet and atherosclerosis. Being a Norwegian, he viewed with a jaundiced eye the report of Ancel Keys and his co-workers that high dietary fat was the single most important cause of atherosclerotic heart disease. Keys (1953) cited the correlation observed between fat intake and death rates from degenerative heart disease in Japan, Italy, Sweden, England and Wales, Canada, Australia, and the United States. Cato believed that in his native Norway, no close relationship existed between fat intake and mortality rate. My observations coincided with those of Gudbrandsen in that my Norwegian family, at least what I knew of them, were high fat consumers, but early death by cardiac disease was not one of their many problems. Using data from the same source as Keys, Gudbrandsen selected seven different countries similar in culture and longevity—Norway, the Netherlands, German Federal Republic, Switzerland, Austria, Israel, and Chile. Gudbrandsen obtained the exact reverse of Keys' results (Figure 12), in that high fat intake seemed to protect against atherosclerotic disease.

Obviously, no firm conclusions can be drawn from either Keys' or Gudbrandsen's data. The data on overall diet apparently were not corrected for total caloric intake. Furthermore, many other risk factors were not considered, factors that are now being better defined. When the discrepancies in the diagnostic habits in the countries utilized by Keys (1953) and data from 22 other countries are included, the rank correlation coefficient of heart disease with dietary fat as a percentage of total calories is not significant. A source of error and obfuscation is that the values used for fat consumption are not the amount of fat eaten, but fat available for consumption. This causes error because much fat is trimmed from meat before cooking, and much of the fat on cooked meat is not eaten (Gudbrandsen, 1961). A further error occurs when documenting the fat *consumed* versus blood lipid levels. A lack of correlation between fat intake and coronary heart disease mortality was also observed in England and the Scandinavian countries during World War II (Hipsley, 1958; Gudbrandsen, 1961).

In England the best correlation existed between mortality from coronary heart disease and the number of radio and television licenses, with a good correlation between heart disease and the number of motor vehicles (see Gudbrandsen, 1961).

A historical perspective might help us understand this complex and costly medical problem in this country. The lifestyle and present diet of human beings is really a recent innovation. Our diet differs markedly in composition from any consumed by wild animals or early people. Our present system of nutrition may go back only about 8,000 years, to the time when some people changed from food gathering to food production. This change led to increased consumption of certain products, including increased intake by some people of meat, dairy products, eggs, and breads, the so-called more luxurious items, described in the Bible as "fat of the land." Increased heart disease may have accompanied this modification in the diet and manner of living, although we admittedly have little data on the incidence of heart disease 8,000 years ago. We do know that Egyptian mummies show evidence of atherosclerosis. Untold resources have been expended trying to determine the causative agents, prevention, and control of this disease complex. The study of risk factors still represents a prodigious investment of scientific talent.

Some studies have focused on heart disease in animals, especially in laboratory animals and in companion animals that share our diet and lifestyle (Kritchevsky, 1974). Cardiovascular disease in dogs and cats living under "normal" family conditions differs from that in people. Dogs (which have been the most studied of the family pets) suffer from congenital heart disease, including valvular problems and cardiomyopathies, but not atherosclerosis. A parvovirus also causes a cardiomyopathy, which may result in sudden death (Ott, personal communication, 1979).

Of more significance in this discussion are canine degenerative heart diseases, for example, muscle degeneration leading ultimately to valvular insufficiency and other valvular problems. It is estimated that by 8 to 9 years of age, at least half of certain breeds of dogs will have some type of cardiac lesion (not atherosclerosis). Most of these diseases will not cause a serious problem, but if the dogs live long enough they will experience gradual deterioration. Most of the dog's heart conditions can be compensated for, so they ultimately die from other causes (Ott, personal communication, 1979;Miller, personal communication, 1979). Our late dog Charlie, whom I refer to as Great Reluctance,[1] lived to be 16 years old, the

---

[1] I called him Great Reluctance because of my wife's concern that I am away from home so much. We found this stray dog for my wife so that whenever I went on a trip I could leave my wife with Great Reluctance.

equivalent in many respects to 80 years in people (Table 2), suffered from nonbacterial endocardiosis, which involves the valves of the heart. (At death, he also had serious kidney problems among other difficulties.) Periodic administration of aminophylline, and later Quibron,® along with a special prescription diet, made Charlie feel like a young dog for a time, charging up and down the hills of Pullman. But dogs are not a suitable model for studying cardiac disease in people.

Pigs in many respects are excellent models for studying the cardiovascular and other systems (Bustad, 1966; Bustad and McClellan, 1966). Although not many pigs are kept for a life span, those that survive have been very useful indeed (Luginbuhl, 1966). Pigs are subject to a number of naturally occurring cardiovascular diseases, such as atherosclerosis, bacterial endocarditis, cardiomyopathy, cerebrovascular accidents, arteriosclerosis, and panarteritis (Detweiler, 1966; Engelhardt, 1966; Maaske et al., 1966; Rowsell et al., 1966). Some nonhuman primates, too, are useful models, as Montagna described in his Wesley Spink lectures in 1975 (Montagna, 1976), and many others have championed (Clarkson et al., 1976, 1979; Baba et al., 1979; Bowden, 1979; and Bowden and Jones, 1979).

The selection and utilization of many small animals and birds as models for studying coronary heart disease has been criticized. There are great advantages for utilizing some of these animals, especially for preliminary studies, because the experiments can be done in a short time (see Vesselinovitch, 1979). One must recognize that if one were to restrict one's efforts to long-term studies on nonhuman primates, one could only do one or two studies in a scientific lifetime, especially if the animal selected were old world monkeys or apes. Some people say one should not use nonhuman primates, but human subjects, restricting the studies to volunteers and prisoners, since they would be better models. This is ethically unacceptable. Also, the human subject is a diverse, out-bred being whose variability almost defies comprehension. An associate, Charles Leathers, stated "If one can bridge the philosophical gap to accept nonhuman primates as appropriate animal models of human disease, then the jump to include other orders of animal life as models is across a mere crevice."

Many have suggested that we need to select a specimen as a test animal or model from the natural state and use it as our basis of study. Naturally occurring arterial lesions have been observed in nonhuman primates living in the wild. But these lesions are typically fibrous rather than fatty, and the secondary complications, especially myocardial infarction and cerebral arterial lesions, are essentially nonexistent. In several parts of the world, people live in much the same way as feral animals; they consume a low fat diet, are very active physically, are nonsmokers, and many are never overweight. Such populations also have insignificant lesions and would not be good candidates for models. These people also add some credence to the belief that atherosclerosis is a disease of "civilizations and industrialization."

Experience strongly suggests that we should stop searching for a nonhuman primate or other species living in the wild with a high incidence of atherosclerosis of the type seen in people in the Western world. Probably no such animal is available today and even if it were, it might not be an appropriate model (Leathers, personal communication, 1979).

Table 6 summarizes characteristics of various animal models for atherosclerosis in people.

RISK FACTORS FOR ATHEROSCLEROSIS

One of the most instructive studies of risk factors in coronary heart disease is the Framingham study. It was designed to determine the factors that influenced the development of coronary heart disease in an adult population consisting of representative samples of over 5,000 people 30 to 62 years old and clinically free of any CHD when the experiment began. The various risk factors examined included diabetes, estrogens, and other hormonal factors, a family history of early atherosclerosis, hypertension, personality factors, physical inactivity, prostaglandins, and smoking of cigarettes. Among

Table 6. Characteristics of Various Animal Models for Atherosclerosis

	Chicken	Pigeon (White Carneau)	Rabbit	Rat	Dog	Pig	Rhesus	Baboon
Appears spontaneously when young	Yes	Yes, some strains	No	No	No	Yes	±Yes	±Yes
Readily induced physiologically	Yes	Yes	Yes	No	No	Yes	Yes	Yes
Sufficient blood available for analysis	Yes	Yes	Yes	For most studies	Yes	Yes	Yes	Yes
Blood lipid patterns similar to human		No	No, but adaptable	No		±Yes	Yes	Yes
Lesions resemble human	Yes, somewhat	Yes, somewhat	Depends on regimen	No	Disease in abdomen	Yes, uncomplicated	Yes, uncomplicated	Yes, uncomplicated
Early changes—proliferating small muscles in intima	Yes	Yes	Depends on regimen	No	No	Yes	Yes	Yes
Advanced plaques evolve with complications	Rarely	Yes (aorta)	Moderate, with time	No	Difficult	Difficult	Rarely reported	Rarely reported
Hemorrhage	No	Yes	Not common	No	Rare	Rare	No	No
Ulceration	No	No	Yes	No	Rare	Rare	Yes	Yes
Necrosis	Yes	Yes	Yes	No	No	Yes	Yes	Yes
Calcification	Not common	Yes	Not common	No	No	Yes	Yes	Yes
Mural thrombosis	Not common	No	Not common	Special	No	Few	Rare	Rare

Table 6 —*Continued*

	Chicken	Pigeon (White Carneau)	Rabbit	Rat	Dog	Pig	Rhesus	Baboon
Infarction	Not common	No	Yes	Special	None by diet alone	Few	Few	Few
Small arteries and aorta involved	Yes	Yes (aorta) ±No (small arteries)	Depends on diet	Yes	Yes	Yes	Yes	Yes
General lipid storage	Yes	No	Depends on diet	Yes	Yes	No	Depends on diet	Depends on diet
Animal large enough	Yes	For some procedures	Yes	No	Yes	Yes	Yes	Yes

these, it appeared that diabetes, a family history of early atherosclerosis, hyperlipidemia, hypertension, and smoking increased incidence and prevalence of atherosclerosis. A combination of the various risk factors greatly increased the probability of cardiovascular disease. It was observed, for example, that the probability of a cardiovascular event occurring within an 8-year period increased from 2% when no risk factors were present to about 50% when risk factors were present (Kannel and Gordon, 1969; see also Hazzard, 1976).

The risk factors are examined below in alphabetical order, with emphasis given to those risk factors for which the most data exist in animals and/or those aspects most familiar to me.

Diabetes   Diabetes mellitus is independent of and also an additive to other risk factors such as hyperlipidemia and hypertension, probably because diabetes affects the microcirculation, producing abnormalities in small coronary vessels as well as major arteries. Atherosclerosis usually occurs at an earlier age and with higher frequency in diabetics. Coronary heart disease incidence is two or three times higher in diabetics than in nondiabetics, and diabetic females are not protected from coronary heart disease during child-bearing years as are nondiabetics (Wilson, personal communication, 1979). Relatively little work has been done on the development of atherosclerosis in spontaneously diabetic animals, since appropriate animal models are in short supply. At Washington State University we have a model for juvenile diabetes in the Keeshond (Kramer, 1977), but we have not observed them for a sufficient period of time to determine if atherosclerosis will develop. Atherosclerosis has been described in the diabetic spiny mouse (Renold et al., 1968). Spontaneously diabetic Black Celebes apes manifest significant atherosclerotic disease, but these animals are in limited supply (Howard, 1973, 1975; Montagna, 1976).

Family History   Those with a positive family history of hypertension, hyperlipidemia, or diabetes, along with an "atherogenic promoting" diet and lifestyle, may show an incidence of coronary heart disease three times greater than those with no such history (Slack and Nevin, 1968). It has been shown that men with a dominantly inherited family history of hypercholesterolemia have a 15-fold increase in risk, and 50% of those with hypercholesterolemia die of coronary heart disease before age 60 (Slack, 1969). Such groups should be the appropriate ones on which to concentrate our efforts, rather than an entire population (Slack and Nevin, 1968; Sokolow and McIlroy, 1979).

Within and between animal species, we observe a variety of responses relative to incidence, lesion distribution, prevalence, and severity of coronary heart disease. Limits on experimental, especially genetic, manipulation of people cause us to rely on these animal models for study. Many years ago Clarkson et al. (1959) noted that the pattern of atherosclerosis in pigeons varied between breeds. Their work also provided special substrains for study of genetic factors. They described white Carneau pigeons that developed spontaneous atherosclerotic lesions that resembled those in people. Interestingly, the serum cholesterol levels of the white Carneau pigeons were no higher than those of other pigeon strains free of atherosclerosis, suggesting a genetic component. In nonhuman primates, squirrel monkeys are of special interest because hyporesponders and hyperresponders to cholesterol-containing diets were identified; by selective breeding, strains were developed having these metabolic characteristics (Lofland et al., 1970). In swine, Rapacz et al. (1977) suggested that by selecting a single sex and similar genotypes, one could obtain relatively uniform plasma low-density lipoprotein (LDL) concentrations in response to certain fatty acids.

Hormonal Estrogen Factors   Women who receive exogenous estrogens have a 20% greater high density lipoprotein (HDL) cholesterol concentration than those not taking these compounds (Gordon et al., 1977a, b). The significance of this is not fully understood. We should note that HDL cholesterol, considered protective against heart attacks, is higher in women than in men. The data in animals are limited, and direct species extrapolation may be possible in only a few higher primates.

Hyperlipidemia   Hyperlipidemia is thought to increase atherosclerosis because of the increased deposits of lipid in the vascular wall caused by high plasma concentration. People with lipid disorders have a high risk of coronary disease if they have hypercholesterolemia. In fact, 85% of these subjects (over four times the normal population) may show myocardial infarction by the age of 60 (Slack, 1969; see also Kritchevsky, 1978).

HDLs are proving one of the more exciting areas of research at the present time. Unfortunately, data on HDL are something less than definitive. However, considerable evidence indicates that the risk of heart attack increases as blood levels of HDL decrease and that low HDL concentrations are a risk factor independent of other known risk factors, including high levels of LDL. Results from the Framingham study indicate that for every decrease in HDL of 5 mg/dl of blood below the average of 45 mg/dl, the risk of heart disease increases 25% (Marx, 1979; Castelli et al., 1977; Kannel et al., 1971, 1979). How to raise HDL cholesterol is of great current interest. Exercising, reducing body weight, increasing alcohol consumption, and being female may raise the HDL cholesterol, but some of these may not be practical, feasible, or recommended. With regard to alcohol, Leathers and associates (1978) found in *Macaca nemestrina* that the severity of coronary artery atherosclerosis may be moderated by ethanol through decreased LDL and coronary artery lumen stenosis and increased HDL. Related studies in people showed that daily intake of small (less than 2 oz) amounts of alcohol was inversely related to coronary death (Hennekens et al., 1979). Caution must be exercised in recommending a therapeutic modality for alcohol, for even small amounts of alcohol consumed by some people can lead to alcoholism.

Of the two principal HDLs reported, HDL2 and HDL3, the HDL3 appears to be associated with protection. Some recent studies by Miller and Miller (1975) and Gordon et al. (1977a,

b) indicate that a decrease in HDL is considerably more important than an increase in LDL or total cholesterol in the development of atherosclerosis. HDL may contribute to the absorption of cholesterol from peripheral tissue, including scavenging of the arterial walls, and movement to the liver where it undergoes biotransformation and excretion. It is important to point out that a dynamic dimension exists among these components because the elements described change as a function of diet and other factors (Munoz et al., 1979; Nichols et al., 1976). Many studies are underway to establish more definitively the function of HDL and other lipids (Brunzell et al., 1978; Glomset, 1979, 1980; see also Andras and Hazzard, 1979; and Mahley et al., 1978).

Glomset (1979, 1980) cautions us about excess optimism about HDL until we know more. HDL obviously has an important role in cholesterol transport; it may contribute to cholesterol balance in the arterial wall. If HDL does remove cholesterol from the arterial wall, most of it may be transferred from HDL to very low density lipoprotein (VLDL) and LDL rather than removed directly by the liver. Studies can not be restricted to finding what increases and what decreases HDL; what is important is its relationship to lipid metabolism, other organ systems, and disease generally and the comparative metabolic parameters in various species.

It is known that HDL falls during pregnancy in several species including macaques (Sackett, personal communication, 1977) but not in people or in the great apes (Glomset, 1980). This suggests that some of our studies on HDL for understanding the situation in people may necessarily be done in a restricted number of expensive species.

Relative to work on nonhuman primates, it was interesting to note that pigtail macaques in limited numbers, whose ages were not known precisely, showed an increase in HDL (high density lipoprotein) cholesterol and LCAT (lecithin: cholesterol acyltransferase) and a decrease in low density lipoprotein (LDL). These changes observed with increasing age may have been a reflection of the selection of survivorship, i.e., the pigtail macaques who lived the longest had high HDL and LCAT and low LDL, and those that didn't died sooner.

At this state of our knowledge, it is premature to state how HDL may protect against atherosclerosis; if you have high amounts in your plasma, just be happy that you have it unless it is elevated because of alcoholism or high intake of chlorinated hydrocarbon pesticides (Carlson and Kolmodin-Hedman, 1977).

Hypertension   Hypertension is considered the most common and most important risk factor in atherosclerosis (Sokolow and McElroy, 1979). One of the principal concerns with hypertension is that it increases the filtration of lipids from plasma to the lining cells of the vessels. Hypertension, along with hyperlipidemia, may result in injury to the intima leading to the proliferation of smooth muscle cells in the media. Increased susceptibility to injury from sheer force and lateral wall pressure, too, may be important. Deming (1975) stated that although diet and serum cholesterol are important, they are much more important if associated with high blood pressure and high estrogen than with low blood pressure and high estrogen. He went on to say that the evidence is absolute: The frequency of cardiac infarction correlates with blood pressure. (Stroke frequency also correlates with blood pressure, and in both of these instances, there is better correlation than with any other risk factor except age.)

The mortality due to coronary heart disease has fallen almost 40% since 1970 and is continuing to decline (Clarkson, personal communication, 1979). This happy turn of events may be due in large part to antihypertensive treatments, many of them developed by drug firms in recent years. In view of this remarkable achievement, it seems appropriate to review the progress made, as well as some interesting history. The relationship between blood pressure and incidence of cardiovascular disease was established just 40 years ago by Clawson (1941). More recent data on four million people and 102,000 deaths by the Build and Blood Pressure Study for the Society of Actuaries (Lew, 1959) showed that life expectancy in both sexes at all ages varied inversely with the arterial blood pressure. Data from this study also showed that with a modest elevation of blood pressure from 148/93 to 177/102, the probability of a person sustaining a cardiac infarct before the age of 40 increased 3.6 times, and the probability of having a stroke went up 15 times.

Data from the Framingham study (and others) have confirmed the relationship between mortality rate and blood pressure. This study also showed a close correlation between blood pressure and cardiac infarction and even a closer one with cerebral infarction. In a 14-year follow-up on the Framingham population, cholesterol was credited with an important role in coronary heart disease, but the research workers stressed that the dominant role was blood pressure in all the various areas of cardiovascular "outcomes." For cerebral infarction or coronary heart disease in older women, one could discriminate using only systolic blood pressure about as accurately as when using all three measurements (i.e., systolic blood pressure, cholesterol, and body weight).

The complex relationships existing between blood pressure and the risk factors of age, sex, cholesterols, smoking, and diabetes are impressive. Some of them correlate with each other and with atherosclerosis. The event that takes place to produce infarction is hemorrhage and thrombosis and appears to be influenced by other factors. The events probably would not occur without a damaged vessel wall. The hemorrhage that occurs is made more likely when arterial pressure is particularly high.

Correlation exists between age and most of the risk factors, including blood pressure, blood cholesterol, diabetes, and possibly smoking (Deming, 1975). The apparent correlation between serum cholesterol and atherosclerosis may result from their dependency on blood pressure. Work in rats in which blood pressure was raised by various means resulted in an increase in the amount of cholesterol (and also the serum cholesterol) in the liver and the whole animal. Through both in vivo and in vitro studies, it was shown that hypertensive rats synthesize cholesterol in the liver and aorta more rapidly than do nonhypertensive controls. The difference in the cholesterol metabolism was not a direct result of the pressure but of the change in the tissues previously brought about by increased blood pressure. This would suggest that blood pressure affects the arterial wall and the serum cholesterol independently.

Decreasing the blood pressure of the hypertensive with a variety of agents does result in decreased serum cholesterol. Abnormal elevation of serum cholesterol in many species may increase atherogenesis. It has been clearly shown that the amount of cholesterol in the arterial wall is independent of serum cholesterol and is correlated more with blood pressure. In some rat studies, it was noted that aortic cholesterol did not change when an atherogenic diet increased serum cholesterol from 82 to 1,257 mg percent. Hypertension, however, did increase the aortic cholesterol and raised the serum cholesterol slightly. The presence of changes in the aortic wall induced by hypertension, diet, and its attendant hypercholesterolemia had a remarkable effect on aortic cholesterol. The locations of the lesions are a function of that pressure. At the point where pressure and turbulence are maximum and external support to the vessel is minimum, the greatest effect is seen on the vessel walls. In an experiment using rats, cross circulation was established so that cholesterol levels were equal. A clip placed on the renal artery of one rat established hypertension, and that rat experienced infarct of the myocardium. The conclusion of a series of studies was that the effect of blood pressure on atherogenesis was not dependent on the effect of blood pressure on serum cholesterol.

Blood pressure causes an increase in diameter of the aorta, which is accompanied by increases in collagen, elastin, and mucopolysaccharides, oxygen consumption, atheroma, and, most important according to Deming (1975), the smooth muscle. In fact, Deming feels the increase in smooth muscle accounts for all the others. Deming also recalls work that indicated smooth muscle hypertrophy itself might be the crucial factor in vascular degeneration and atherosclerosis. The work of Deming and associates indicates that the principal cell of the artery is the muscle cell, which serves a multiple function (see Wolinsky, 1973). It contracts and secretes extracellular proteins, collagen, elastin, and mucopolysaccharides, as well as cholesterol. It is present in the subendothelium, as well as the media, and is the major, if not only, cellular element in the plaque. This cell responds to a number of stimuli, and high blood pressure provokes proliferation of the cells; lipids may also stimulate the cells. Estrogen treatment, according to Deming (1975), has an inhibitory effect on aortic wall response to hypertension.

Platelets and Prostaglandins   Recently Gingrich and Hoak (1979) stated that the decade of the 1970s could be described as the period of prostaglandins and endothelium. I believe the next few years might be aptly called the era of the platelet and prostaglandin. Prostaglandins, the local hormones synthesized by most tissues, have become important subjects for study in the very recent past. It is known that a number of different prostaglandins are formed from the enzymatic breakdown of arachidonic acid, an unsaturated fatty acid. These degradation products are important because they may promote vasodilation or platelet aggregation (thromboxanes) or antiplatelet aggregation (prostacyclins) that could determine whether aggregation occurs. Agglutination of the platelets is considered an important element in the development of atherosclerotic plaques. In the absence of an antiplatelet aggregating substance, the prostacyclins, platelet aggregation may be enhanced. Aspirin is thought to inhibit the early stages of arachidonic acid breakdown, and it is for that reason some people use it. It may be helpful in improving coronary blood flow (Sokolow and McIlroy, 1979).

This discussion of atherosclerosis has described the use of animal models for defining the syndrome, with the object of prevention, control, and treatment. An interesting application of some unusual models to help unravel the "puzzle of the platelets" in atherosclerosis is exemplified by studies in cattle, mink, and cats at Washington State University that manifest the Chédiak-Higashi syndrome, and pigs in Minnesota that manifest von Willebrand's disease. A common characteristic of these two diseases is platelet dysfunction. Since platelets appear to be involved in the atherosclerotic process both terminally in thrombosis and in the initiating events, I thought it would be useful to discuss briefly the application of these unusual animal models.

Meyers and associates (1979a, b) have shown that animals with Chédiak-Higashi syndrome have abnormal bleeding that can be attributed to impaired platelet function, which results from a deficiency of compounds stored within certain platelet granules. As a consequence, these platelets have a reduced ability to aggregate and secrete platelet factors. With this defect, animals with Chédiak-Higashi syndrome offer the scientific community a unique opportunity to study atherosclerosis and its ramifications. In addition, since the platelet defect prevents the formation of an effective thrombus, we have an animal model in which to develop new and viable means of controlling thrombosis.

Pigs with von Willebrand's disease are an animal model where platelet-surface interaction is defective. Fuster and Bowie (1978) have used this model to determine if experimental animals known to have impaired platelet function are less prone to the development of atherosclerosis. They found that, unlike normal pigs, the pig with von Willebrand's disease was resistant to atherosclerosis. This important finding provides the first evidence in an experimental animal (where the platelet or the animal had not been pharmacologically modified) that platelets are involved in the initiation of atherosclerosis. Furthermore, Ross et al. (1974) have shown that platelets contain factor(s) that promote smooth muscle proliferation. With damage to the vessel lining (the endothelium), platelets attach to the arterial surface. With the release of these factor(s), smooth muscle proliferation is stimulated, and this represents the first step in the atherosclerosis lesion.

By learning more about how platelets react and function.

we may be able to modify their response, thereby aborting the initial event, as well as possibly preventing the terminal event, thrombosis. We hope these models will help us define pathways of platelet activation in many animals, and understand basic properties of platelets. We hope, too, that this information will assist in developing improved antiplatelet and antiaggregating agents. These agents are important in preventing atherosclerosis and thrombosis, and in developing and maintaining artificial surfaces used in an assortment of prosthetic devices in the cardiovascular system, including heart valves, bypasses, artificial hearts and heart assist devices, blood vessels, and catheters. The benefits of this knowledge can be great, especially for the elderly.

Physical Inactivity   Lack of exercise is often cited as one of the risk factors in atherosclerosis. A sedentary life and the associated obesity that usually results appear to predispose people to hypertension and diabetes. Since inactive people usually have reduced luminal area in the coronary and other vessels, their chance of survival following a myocardial infarction is considered less than that of other people. The value of exercise has been actively promoted recently to prevent coronary heart disease, but all persons who have cardiac disease may not be helped by exercise. Relative to animals, Fox (1933) observed that those animals who prance, run, jump, and climb the most are least affected by cardiovascular disease, while those who are rather quiet, placid animals—the bovine, the parrot, and domestic ducks—exhibited the highest incidence of lesions. May (1958) observed that people who had been very active, even physically powerful, individuals but for various reasons had slipped into a sort of muscular retirement appeared to be the most common victims of coronary thrombosis. Paul Dudley White (1958) stated that if everybody paid more attention to the benefit of exercise, there might be less hypertension and coronary heart disease. He had earlier observed that heart disease and blood pressure are less common in those who maintain a habit of exercise and at the same time avoid obesity. Gudbrandsen (1961) noted that many observations seem to support the theory that physical inactivity, combined with high caloric intake, may be the most important single factor in causing atherosclerotic disease. It is noted that countries where coronary heart disease incidence is low are industrially underdeveloped, with a high percentage of the population involved in hard physical labor, with few or no automobiles, radios, or TV sets (Morris and Heady, 1953; Morris and Crawford, 1958; see also Froelicher, 1972).

Many occupational studies seem to support the beneficial effects of physical activity on lowering the incidence of coronary heart disease (Gudbrandsen, 1961; Morris and Crawford, 1958; Morris and Heady, 1953; Morris et al., 1956, 1958; Paffenbarger and Hale, 1975; Wong et al., 1973; see also Froelicher, 1972). In a Swedish study, Biorck and co-workers (1954) observed that 27% of the infarcts in the population were in 9% of the population who were "mental" workers while only 5% of the infarcts were in 33% of the population that had hard labor to perform. Overall, 11% of the total population were doing mental work and suffered 1/3 of the cardiac-infarcts. The Swedish workers all had about the same medical care, irrespective of their social status.

Paffenbarger and Hale (1975) observed that longshoremen who were followed for up to 22 years or to age 75 or death showed that "high" work activity resulted in lower age-adjusted coronary death rates than lower work activity. This protective effect was most noteworthy for the sudden death syndrome (5.6 deaths/10,000 work years for high work activity compared with 20 for moderate activity).

In experimental studies with chicks (Wong et al., 1973; Orma, 1957) and rabbits (Kobernick et al., 1957; Myasnikov, 1958), exercise was associated with a reduction in atherosclerosis. Eckstein (1957) observed that coronary narrowing in dogs stimulated collateral circulation, as did exercise.

For some time we have thought that increased collateral circulation is one chief benefit of exercise, but this issue is under debate (Froelicher, 1972). Sanders et al. (1977, 1978) observed no increase in coronary collaterals after 10 months of endurance exercise training in pigs, a very good model for people. The luminal area of coronary arteries may be enlarged by exercise and the high density lipids seem to be increased with exercise. In fact, these may be the two chief benefits of exercise, besides the feeling of "well-being" that often results. Relative to the higher levels of HDL in runners, this may not be a clear-cut case either, for in a study by Wood at Stanford, the group of runners also were found to smoke less, drink more, and weigh less (Marx, 1979). All three of these factors are consistent with higher HDL levels. Other changes with exercise are increases in skeletal muscle mitochondria and respiratory enzymes, which at least partially account for increased aerobic work capacity (Holloszy, 1971).

Experiments on exercise specifically for the elderly are very limited. Shephard (1978), working with patients who experienced myocardial infarction, noted a good response to progressive long-distance training. For people 60 to 70 years of age, the occasional reports are contradictory and probably reflect the nature of the exercise regimen. Shephard (1978) conducted supervised exercise classes for older people for one hour four times each week for over a year of progressive training. Initial pulse rates of 120/min were achieved, with progression to rates of 140 to 150 with increased fitness. Over an extended period, people training regularly at low intensity achieved gains similar to those of a high intensity group. The elderly in Shephard's study lost more than 3 mm subcutaneous fat over a period of one year. There was also a small increase in lean body mass. Bone calcium in these individuals increased or at least held constant.

If one were to rely on data from exercised rats, one would hesitate to encourage high intensity exercise in the elderly. Regular swimming in rats conferred a small increase in longevity only if it was begun at an early age. If begun after maturity, a decrease in longevity was observed.

Smoking of Cigarettes   Smoking is not a problem in animals except in those we subject to this hazard. The frequency of smoking of cigarettes is exceedingly high in people with atherosclerotic disease. The factors involved are probably associated with carbon monoxide and nicotine. Nicotine elevates plasma norepinephrine, and epinephrine, and it also increases free fatty acid concentrations, blood pressure, pulse rate, and myocardial oxygen consumption. Cigarette smoking induces arrhythmias and appears to promote atherosclerosis. As stated above, heavy smoking is associated with the reduced serum HDL cholesterol (Kannel et al., 1978). The weight of evidence is overwhelming against cigarette smoking. In terms of cost of life and property, it must be the world's worst addiction. Animals should not be subjected to cigarette smoke except under very unusual, experimental circumstances. The one positive note on cigarette smoking is that a year after one quits smoking, risk factors related to smoking and coronary heart disease decrease to those of nonsmokers and the recovery from damage is remarkable.

REGRESSION OF ATHEROSCLEROSIS

A significant drop in mortality rates due to atherosclerotic heart disease during World Wars I and II was noted in some European countries. It was suggested that the disease might be reversible through modification of diet and lifestyle (Katz and Stamler, 1953; Katz et al., 1958). Some workers reported regression of lesions noted at necropsy; such regression also was noted in functional and angiographic evaluations of coronary and peripheral circulation in people following severe restrictions of food intake, hormone therapy for cancer, chronic wasting disease, ileal bypass, drug therapy, and other measures reviewed by Wissler and Vesselinovitch (1975). In view of these observations, it seemed worthwhile to pursue definitive studies in experimental animals to evaluate the feasibility of various procedures for effecting regression of atherosclerotic plaques.

Some interesting studies on regression have used pigs and

nonhuman primates. Armstrong et al. (1970) and Armstrong and Megan (1972) fed rhesus monkeys an atherogenic diet that produced serious lesions; they noted remarkable improvement after a 40-month period of feeding either low fat and low cholesterol rations or a high corn oil and low cholesterol diet. The improvement involved a substantial decrease in luminal narrowing in all main coronary arteries of the severely affected rhesus monkeys with serum cholesterol levels that averaged about 140 mg percent. There also was an absolute decrease in collagen and elastin content of the vessels.

Other studies, chiefly on monkeys, reveal regression using low fat and cholesterol free, or low fat and corn oil diets. Wissler and Vesselinovitch (1975) used coconut oil instead of butter, which has greater atherogenicity and accelerates the atherosclerosis process. Some of the animals were killed after 18 months and others were fed low fat and low cholesterol rations, with added W-1372 (n-γ-Phenylpropyl-N-Benzyloxy Acetamide — an anticholesteremia agent) in the ration of one group. Both groups exhibited significant regression of aortic lesions, but the drug did not produce an added effect over the diet. The narrowing of the vessels was reduced up to one-half the degree of narrowing before therapy. There was also a reduction in the aortic cholesterol and collagen (see Malinov et al., 1976).

Another study using monkeys involved 12 months of feeding a low fat diet alone or in combination with cholestyramine (a bio-salt sequestering agent at levels of 25 g/kg ration). The low fat regimen, with or without cholestyramine, evidenced the greatest regression (Wissler and Vesselinovitch, 1975; Vesselinovitch et al., 1974). In the latter study, the severe atherosclerotic lesions in rabbits were remarkably reduced in size by a therapeutic regimen of oxygen administration, low fat diet, and either estrogen or cholestyramine therapy.

Clarkson et al. (1973) conducted a comprehensive study in the avian species using white Carneau pigeons. A cholesterol free diet after a year of an atherogenic one resulted in a marked decrease in free and esterified cholesterol in plaques, in coronary artery lumen stenosis, and in frequency of myocardial infarction.

Some workers observed regression of advanced aortic atherosclerosis induced by an atherogenic diet and mechanical injury by balloon catheters in swine fed a high mash diet low in fat for 14 months (Daoud et al., 1976; Fritz et al., 1976). If these results can be extrapolated to people, the prognosis for possible regression of atherosclerosis with strict controlled diet is a real possibility.

In an important long-term study, Clarkson and associates (1979) fed an atherogenic diet to the monkeys for 19 or 38 months, and then grouped the animals to determine any difference in regression between animals kept at two different levels of serum cholesterol. They found a beneficial effect on the artery, that is, more regression, with plasma cholesterol levels of 200 compared with the 300 mg/dl group. There appeared to be a therapeutic benefit of a 100 mg/dl difference. Their study also suggested that long-term induced lesions regress less than short-term ones. A surprising finding was that the most susceptible animals of the group were little affected by the additional time they were fed the atherogenic diet, while those in the middle range were the most affected. If their results could be applied to the clinical situation, therapeutic intervention in people, to be effective, should be done by age 30. However, some studies have demonstrated that the average reduction in serum cholesterol concentrations by use of "prudent diets" is on the order of 10 to 15%, and whether such a modest reduction in serum cholesterol would result in significant regression of arterial plaques remains to be seen.

More recently, a sucrose polyester has been used to reduce serum cholesterol. This compound consists of sucrose and long chains of fatty acids and has the appearance and physical properties of the usual dietary fats but is neither absorbed nor digested (Fallat et al., 1976). Dogs and rats have been used to study its effects. When it was incorporated in the diet, replacing as much as 90% of the dietary fat, it was effective in reducing the total and low-density lipoprotein cholesterol by 15% and 17%, respectively, when the animals were fed high cholesterol diets. But it was ineffective in patients with familial hypercholesterolemia. When fed to people, it did not seem to cause any substantial gastrointestinal discomfort, although it did decrease absorption of some soluble compounds in the diet, including vitamins A and E. The use of a liquid sucrose polyester would have several advantages over the cholesterol binding resins or the phytosterols because it can be readily incorporated into many routine foodstuffs or substituted for the conventional dietary fats. Its long-term safety, of course, will have to be determined by prolonged feeding. Clarkson (personal communication, 1979) stated that when sucrose polyester is included with dietary cholesterol, it lowers plasma lipids. In contrast, if animals are relatively nonresponsive to dietary cholesterol, it has little effect; it seems to affect a particular metabolic group, namely, the one responsive to dietary cholesterol.

A final note on regression relates to surgical intervention pioneered at the University of Minnesota by Buckwald and co-workers (1975). They utilized a partial ileal bypass in patients with severe hypercholesterolemia and atherosclerosis. Sequential coronary arteriograms showed no progression of the disease in over half of the patients over a three-year period. Thirteen percent had definite evidence of regression of the coronary atherosclerosis. These workers also noted a large decrease in serum cholesterol, as well as a reduction in the area of atherosclerosis, within one year after instituting a cholesterol lowering diet, drugs, and exercise for heart attack patients. The evaluation was based on a panel method of unbiased radiological interpretations of sequential coronary arteriograms. Blankenhorn (1977) and also DePalma et al. (1972, 1977) developed useful methods for evaluating regression.

Several questions on regression remain unanswered. One of the most important is whether the reduction of the plaque and the fibrous replacement of it might in some cases be worse than the original disease. Critical to people my age, and especially those who are older, is whether these therapeutic regimens can be effective on 50-year-old plaques. Perhaps for people my age, the regimens are like chicken soup—they probably won't do any harm and might do some good (see Prichard, 1974). Many of us look forward to the completion of the HEW-Multiple Risk Factor Intervention Trial scheduled for 1982. This study is assessing the effectiveness of measures to reduce elevated blood cholesterol, high blood pressure, and cigarette smoking in preventing first heart attacks and reducing death rates from cardiovascular diseases in many thousands of men age 35 to 57.

SPECIFIC RECOMMENDATIONS FOR
PREVENTING ATHEROSCLEROSIS

Relative to recommendations on diet and lifestyle, the regimen established should be familiar, feasible, fundable, and readily facilitated. A reasonable and palatable diet should be developed for each person (Weg, 1978; Connor and Connor, 1972; Sirtori et al., 1973). Moderate measures should be replaced only if they fail to elicit necessary reductions in body weight, high blood pressure, and dangerously high levels of blood lipids. The regimen should be directed at overcoming inadequacies and excesses in dietary and living routines. Relative to nutritional aspects and hypertension, this, of course, is in part dependent on the etiology and nature of the disease. Generally, it is well to restrict sodium intake. It isn't enough just to reduce salt intake if one is trying to reduce sodium intake for hypertension. Soups and condiments contain much sodium. Catsup, monosodium glutamate, sodium bicarbonate, and sodium nitrate and nitrate (in preserved foods) are common sources of sodium and appear in substantial amounts in processed foods (Kolata, 1979). Caloric intake should be restricted to prevent obesity. Excessive alcohol is contraindicated, and attention should be given to any carbohydrate intolerance. A diet that would reduce plasma triglycerides and cholesterol if patients have hyperlipidemias would seem prudent.

Unfortunately, I cannot make any more specific recommendations on nutrition except to say that many interesting studies are underway. A recent example is a study on vitamin E, a controversial issue, which showed that this vitamin inhibited atherogenesis in rabbits (Wilson et al., 1978). (Summary recommendations on nutrition appear in the Afterword.)

For those who have a familial history of atherosclerosis, during middle age the following recommendations may be appropriate. Fruit should replace desserts containing high amounts of sucrose. Dietary fiber may be very helpful (Jenkins et al., 1975). A diet of about 30% or less fat is more reasonable than some diets that have up to 60%. Oils that are low in transfatty acids are recommended; until we learn more about transfatty acids, I refrain from using material high in transfatty acids (in this regard, I use butter, but not very much of it, in preference to margarine, and for my tea and postum, I use milk instead of cream substitutes, which contain over 50% transfatty acid). Only moderate amounts of meat should be consumed, and this should be lean meat preferably prepared by boiling or steaming, avoiding prolonged high temperatures. All meat should be trimmed of excess fat. At this stage of our knowledge, these recommendations seem appropriate for those who are hypertensive or have hypercholesterolemia in excess of 250 mg/100 ml, and for those who are obese. The goal should be adapting a diet to each person; it is important to consider individual variation before making sweeping recommendations (Ahrens, 1979).

Moderation in activities should be emphasized, and an animal companion recommended if the patient is in a position to have one. A low intensity exercise regimen appears to be more beneficial to the health and well-being of many elderly than does a high intensity regimen. It may be of special benefit to the diabetic (Gonzalez, 1979). I find a low intensity exercise program very important to me: By this I mean walking or riding a bicycle a couple of miles a day up and down hills and walking up and down all stairs. Physical exercise of 20 to 30 minutes a day, at least three or four times a week to raise the heart rate to 120-150 (depending on age) appears reasonable. Frustrating elements in a person's life should be addressed and positive attempts made to diminish or relieve them. Smoking should be eliminated. The best advice was given by my son, a cardiologist, when he told me to be moderate in all things except moderation (L. B. Bustad, personal communication, 1979).

Cancer

Most people in North America consider cancer to be the most awesome and challenging problem facing science and society today. The great fear that the word engenders stems from the enormous personal consequences of cancer for both those afflicted and their families (Busch, 1979; Bustad, 1973; Bustad et al., 1976). Although cancer causes only about one-half as many deaths each year in the United States as cardiovascular disease, many people with whom I have discussed this subject would prefer to die from a heart attack than cancer, if given that choice.

Few people today underestimate the problem of cancer. The number of new patients diagnosed approaches 700,000 each year, with more than a million patients under treatment and over 350,000 deaths per year. It is estimated that cancer costs the American public somewhere between 20 and 30 billion dollars annually. Most of us have lost a good friend in the recent past because of cancer or know someone undergoing therapy or recently diagnosed as having cancer.

What many people fail to realize is that cancer is not just one disease. There are over 100 types of cancer (see Clark and Rauscher, 1977). Of special importance to the elderly is that many cancers are considered controllable, even curable, and there have been marked increases in survival. The mortality and incidence of the various cancers varies considerably (Silverberg, 1979) (Table 7). In people as well as in many animals with which I have worked, the incidence of cancer in-

Table 7. Estimated Cancer Incidence and Death by Site and Sex for 1979
(modifed from Silverberg, 1979)

Site	Female Incidence	Death	Site	Male Incidence	Death
Breast	27*	19*	Lung	22*	34*
Colon and			Prostrate	17	10
rectum	15	15	Colon and		
Uterus	13	6	rectum	14	12
Lung	8	14	Urinary	10	5
Leukemia and			Leukemia and		
lymphomas	7	9	lymphomas	8	9
Ovary	4	6	Oral	5	3
Urinary	4	3	Pancreas	3	5
Pancreas	3	5	Skin	2	1
Skin	2	1	Other	19	21
Oral	2	1			
Other	15	21			

*Expressed as percentage of those with cancer in United States.

creases with age. Those who are 25 years old now have one chance in 700 of developing cancer by age 30, while those who are 65 years old have one chance in 14 of developing cancer by age 70 (Butler and Gastel, 1979; see Enstrom and Austin, 1978). There is much speculation whether aging and cancer share a common process (Comfort, 1971; Pitot, 1977). One argument is that mutations may be involved in both processes (Butler and Gastel, 1979).

Until recently most people regarded cancer as a mysterious, unpredictable, unavoidable, usually fatal disease. Although cancer is still to a considerable degree mysterious and unpredictable, we realize that many cancers are neither fatal nor unavoidable. The perception that cancer may originate in the activities of people, that it is a "man-made" problem, should stimulate us to understand and avoid it.

John Higginson, founding director of the World Health Organization's International Agency for Research on Cancer, proposed 30 years ago that two-thirds of all cancers had an environmental cause and were, therefore, preventable. On the basis of his studies of epidemiological data such as differences between Africans and Americans, he suggested that most cancers were not due to genetic but to environmental factors, involving the total environment, including air, agricultural practices, behavior, chemicals, culture, diet, and water (Maugh, 1979). But I hesitate to completely discount the genetic and perhaps infectious component.

Although I sympathize with Higginson's views on the complexity of the various factors involved in carcinogenesis, the fact remains that even though we are all exposed to an assortment of carcinogenic agents, comparatively few of us develop cancer. Controlling only carcinogens and mutagens will probably not eradicate very many cancers, for such measures involve only the initiation phase of carcinogenesis. To blame pollution for all our cancers is an oversimplification. We can compare a clean city with a very dirty one and discover the cancer incidence is about the same: it probably depends on the nature of the "dirt" and the length of exposure. We should broaden our examination to include lifestyle, such as behavioral and cultural patterns, and dietary, smoking, and drinking habits (Redmond, 1970; Higginson and Muir, 1979). An evaluation of these, modified from John Higginson's estimates, appears in Figure 13.

Even these rough estimates indicate the relative importance of the various factors. Obviously, diet is a critical factor. Fats, proteins, and vegetable inhibitors all may be important. Caloric and fat intake should be reduced in many people and fiber included in the diet.

The principle classes of carcinogens (which are also mutagens) are viruses, physical agents, and chemicals. A brief review of viruses and physical agents is necessary since the various agents may operate in concert. A chemical may promote a viral carcinogen, or cancer may be induced by a physical agent, e.g., radiation, and promoted by a dietary component or deficiency.

VIRUSES

The first animal tumor virus was described in leukemic chickens by Ellerman and Bang (1908). Since leukemia was

Factor

Diet   oooooooooooooooooooooooooooooooooooooooooo (42)
            xxxxxxxxxxxxxxxxxxxxxxxxx (25)

Tobacco &   oooooooooo (10)
Alcohol   xxxxxxxxxxxxxxxxxxxxxxxxxxxxxxxxxxxxx (35)

Culture &   oooooooooooooooooo (18)
Behavior   xxxxx (5)

Sunlight   oooooooooo (10)
            xxxxxxxxxx (10)

Occupation oo (2)
            xxxxxx (6)

Figure 13. Proportions of cancers due to various factors modified from estimates made by Higginson and
Muir (1979) (females = o and males = x).

not considered a neoplastic disease, this discovery attracted
very little serious attention. Within three years, Peyton Rous
discovered a virus in a solid tumor – a sarcoma in a chicken.
Again, the medical community gave little attention to this
finding. Fortunately, however, Peyton Rous was blessed with
a long life; in fact, he lived long enough to be awarded the
Nobel Prize in 1966 – 55 years after his noteworthy discovery
(Rous, 1911, 1965). Since that time, scientists have isolated
other tumor viruses (RNA type) that cause leukosis and sar-
comas in birds, fibrosarcoma and lymphosarcoma in cats, lymphosarcoma in cattle and sheep, and tumors in a variety of
laboratory animals, including nonhuman primates (see Essex,
1979; Essex et al., 1980). I shared the excitement of the
times when my associates in comparative oncology at the
University of California-Davis were the first to discover the
viruses that cause fibrosarcoma in cats and woolly monkeys
and lymphosarcomas in gibbons (apes) (Theilen et al., 1971;
Snyder and Theilen, 1969; Kawakami et al., 1972, 1973,
1975). Herpes viruses (DNA type) that cause Marek's disease

in chickens, lymphomas in some monkeys, and possibly adenomatosis in sheep have also been isolated. They have been implicated in Burkitt's lymphoma, carcinoma of the cervix, and nasopharyngeal carcinoma in Chinese people.

One of the newest developments in virus research is the identification of viral gene products (a protein kinase) that may be able to convert a normal chicken cell into a sarcoma cell. With tumor viruses, only a piece of the original viral DNA or RNA may be in the host cell, perhaps incorporated into the host's genome. It is probable that chemicals can so damage cells that a carcinogenic virus may more readily cause the transformation to cancer. In a way, a cancer is an accident in which many factors unfortunately come together at a particular time.

Vaccination against tumors of viral origin has been successful in at least two instances—Marek's disease of chickens and fibropapillomatosis of cattle. A vaccine is currently being tested for leukemia in cats. Since cancer is, in most instances, a chronic disease with complex and multiple causes, no one vaccine will probably be discovered to prevent the disease. However, cancer virus studies may help us define the mechanism and agents involved in the transformation of normal cells into cancer cells (see Ahuja and Anders, 1977; Gallo, 1977; and Rapp and Reed, 1977).

PHYSICAL AGENTS

Among the carcinogenic physical agents, radiation (ionizing and ultraviolet) has received the most attention. Much of my scientific career has been spent in radiation studies, but the discussion here will touch only the highlights of the subject. The extensive accumulated experimental data on animals and people have furnished a firm basis for assigning exposure limits that permit us to work safely in industries and other areas where ionizing radiation is employed. The exposure of the general public is far below levels at which toxicity would be expected to be manifest. However, exposure to sunlight, with its ultraviolet radiation, can cause cancer as well as redness and serious conditions in certain people and animals exposed to specific plant chemicals containing photosensitizing agents (Scheel, 1973).

Compared with chemical carcinogens, radiation appears inefficient and slow in producing deleterious effects. The significance of many animal experiments involving radiation is that they appear to be applicable to people (Bustad, 1976a). Many of the studies with which I have been involved emphasized feeding radionuclides, which are potential hazards in case of nuclear fallout or nuclear industry contamination events. Dietary constituents were important considerations in such studies. In the case of radioiodine administration, the normal, stable (nonradioactive) iodine content of the diet determined in great part the radioiodine uptake by the thyroid. In fact, sufficient stable iodine could be administered to block any appreciable radioiodine uptake (Bustad et al., 1958).

Chemicals   During my lifetime of 60 years, the number of chemicals has increased phenomenally, to the point where probably upwards of 7 million chemicals are in existence. At least 50,000 chemicals are now of commercial importance in the United States. Every day, two new chemicals enter commerce. Millions of pounds of these chemicals are imported or produced, transported, and used each week. An industrial solvent, 1,2-dichloroethane, which is used in the synthesis of vinyl chloride, is produced in the United States at the rate of 10 billion pounds annually. The pesticide toxaphene is produced at the rate of 100 million pounds annually. Both of these agents have been shown to be carcinogenic for animals (Griesemer, 1979) and are probably carcinogenic for people.

Unfortunately, of the 50,000 chemicals on the market, relatively few have been adequately tested for carcinogenicity. About 7,000 have been at least partially tested, with about 20% of these showing evidence of carcinogenicity (Davis and Magee, 1979). We have enough information to consider 400 of them as animal carcinogens, and up to 35 as human carcinogens. The one chemical proved to be a carcinogen in people, but not animals, is arsenic (Griesemer, 1979).

With this brief introduction you may well ask, "If the headlines suggest that most cancers are caused by chemicals, which ones are doing all the damage?" Unfortunately, many news accounts are exaggerated. Recently it was stated that 60 to 90% of human cancers are environmentally caused (Culliton, 1978; Maugh, 1979). It is important to realize that "environment" refers to all extrinsic factors and includes air, food, water, sunshine, special dietary items, and lifestyle factors, including smoking and alcohol consumption. Since the great proliferation of chemicals in the environment has occurred only in the last two decades, the nature of their impact on the human population will not be known for several years because of the latency required for tumors to be manifested.

A myriad of substances, including naturally occurring ones, may induce tumors in people. The National Academy of Sciences published a 624-page book (NAS-1973) that lists an assortment of agents such as microbial toxins, spices, sweeteners, food lipids, amino acids and peptides, nitrites, nitrates, excesses of vitamins, trace elements, and natural food chemicals. Three of these will be discussed because of the great current interest in them: nitrates, aflatoxins, and saccharin.

Nitrosamine, Nitrate, and Nitrite   The nitrate and nitrite content of food has become a subject of great concern because of reports of carcinogenicity (Fassett, 1973; Issenberg, 1976). Nitrates appear in much of what we eat, including vegetables and cured meat. Nitrate as saltpeter has been added to meat since the dawn of history for preservation and to give it better color and flavor. More recently, we discovered it also prevents the growth of botulinum organisms that produce a deadly toxin (Foster, personal communication, 1978). Nitrate is reduced to nitrite and then to nitric oxide by bacterial action. (This can occur in our intestines.) Nitric oxide reacts with meat pigments to give a characteristic pink color in cured meat. Nitrites may combine with substances called amines forming nitrosamines, which are carcinogenic. Nitrosamines can be formed from nitrite in bacon, especially when it is fried using high temperatures. The basis of much of the concern is that N-nitroso compounds may be produced during processing, storage, and preparation of foods, as well as in the mammalian stomach because of the acid pH there.

After a visit to Homan, China, Kaplan and Tsuchitani (1978) described probable carcinogens in food and feed there. The source of the carcinogen may be a regional dietary staple containing a pickled mixture of vegetables that are stored for up to six months. Moldy corn bread and hot foods were suggested as contributory. The mold that accumulates on the vegetable mulch (and on the cornbread) is eaten. The pH of the pickled mixture is in the range of 3-4, a level at which secondary amines may be converted to nitrosamines. An Ames test of this mixture indicated the presence of mutagens. Chickens in the Honan region receiving table scraps developed carcinomas mainly of the pharyngeal region. However, this was not the first instance of suspected carcinogenesis. The first work reported involved a study on rats that developed liver cancer following feeding of 50 ppm of dimethylnitrosamine (Magee and Barnes, 1956). Since this report over two decades ago, a number of N-nitroso compounds have been identified as experimental carcinogens. These compounds have been shown to induce a variety of tumors in different organ sites depending on the structure of the compound, the species of animal utilized, and the dose and route of administration (Magee and Barnes, 1967). In addition to cancer, acute toxic effects with large doses have been observed. One noteworthy incident occurred in sheep that developed acute liver necrosis after being fed nitrite-preserved fish meal. Some of the sheep died; the meal contained dimethylnitrosamine presumably formed by the reaction of nitrate with free amines (Ender et al., 1964).

No consistent pattern of N-nitroso compounds in cured meats, a commonly cited source, seems evident. Nitrosamines occur sporadically but usually at very low levels.

This inconsistency is not surprising because several factors, many undefined, influence the rates of nitrosation reactions, including catalysts, inhibitors, pH, and temperature. We know, for example, that bacterial action can produce nitrite, a very reactive substance, from nitrate. Bacteria also are implicated in forming N-nitroso compounds, e.g., nitrosamines. Low reaction rates over a period of time can yield substantial N-nitroso compounds during food processing, storage, and preparation. Many compounds that react with nitrates may tend to inhibit the formation of nitrosamines: ascorbic acid (vitamin C) is one of these. Sodium ascorbate at high levels can prevent formation of dimethylnitrosamines during processing of frankfurters. Smoking of cured meats may also block N-nitroso compounds from forming, owing to certain components in smoke (e.g., phenolic components) that react readily with nitrate. Other compounds, including some in the natural environment, may accelerate the formation of N-nitroso compounds, including thiocyanate, which occurs in normal saliva and gastric juice. Formaldehyde also acts to accelerate nitrosation rates; this could be important in long-term storage of certain foods. High temperature can also increase nitrosation. In view of these many factors, it is no wonder sporadic analytical results occur; there are also probably many N-nitroso compounds to which we are exposed of which we are not aware. Far more experimental work needs to be done.

To evaluate the hazards of N-nitroso compounds, one must determine the sources of nitrite and nitrate in foods and in the body. To assign cured meats as the major source of nitrates is unrealistic when one considers the high nitrate level in many other food items such as leafy vegetables, including spinach, lettuce, turnip greens, radishes, beets, celery, and eggplant. In some people, saliva alone may have up to 10 ppm of nitrite. The contribution of cured meats to gastric nitrite is variously estimated at 16 to over 30% (White, 1975), whereas that from saliva is estimated at approximately 70%. Most of this comes from ingested nitrate. The nitrate content of vegetables is dependent on the amount of fertilizer, light intensity, available water, and plant damage. Some water supplies are high in nitrate (they should not exceed 10 ppm) (Wolff and Wasserman, 1972). Nitrate itself is not the principal culprit; reducing it to nitrite (and then to N-nitroso compounds) constitutes the primary hazard. Microbial environments such as might occur in spinach or other damp vegetable matter high in nitrate, or low pH in the stomach contribute to formation of nitrites from nitrates.

Government officials are considering banning the use of nitrates and nitrites in the preservation of meat, but it is well to examine the wisdom and impact of such action. Consideration is also being given to disallowing use of any product containing nitrosamines. Because of the hazards of botulinum toxicity in cured meats (which is prevented by nitrite), it appears unwise to ban nitrates and nitrites until a reasonable and safer substitute is available. A promising one that has been proposed is 0.26% potassium sorbate combined with 40 ppm of nitrite, rather than the 120 ppm nitrite and 550 ppm erythorbate now used.

Since we obtain the majority of our nitrate from sources other than cured meats, the cancer risk probably will not be measurably decreased by eliminating preserved meats (Foster, personal communication, 1978). Furthermore, nitrates are reduced to nitrites in the body and nitrosamines are formed in the body in the absence of preserved meats. It would be prudent to use a variety of meats (and vegetables in the diet) and not depend on preserved meats as the only protein source. Since high temperatures promote nitrosamine formation, prolonged high heat should not be used in the cooking of meats. For example, a radar oven is the preferred way to prepare bacon. In fact, it is recommended that prolonged high temperatures should not be used in preparation of most foods. This recommendation is made because carcinogenic hydrocarbons have been identified in the smoke as well as on the charred material on the surface of smoked or grilled meat (Upton, personal communication, 1979).

Aflatoxins   Aflatoxins serve as a representative of a naturally occurring toxin in many food sources. The two principal aflatoxins are B1 and G1, with their less toxic derivatives being B2 and G2. Aflatoxin B1 is considered by some to be the most potent liver carcinogen for laboratory animals. The aflatoxin story began in England in 1960 in an outbreak of "turkey disease" (Blount, 1961), manifested as an acute liver disease that caused high mortality in turkey poults. The causative agent was traced to rations containing peanut meal contaminated with *Aspergillus flavus* mold. Since that time a massive literature has been developed. We now know that grains may become contaminated during unfavorable growing and harvesting conditions and improper storage. Aflatoxins are also formed by fungi other than *A. flavus*. The aflatoxins are carcinogenic in a wide range of species, and evidence that aflatoxin is carcinogenic was well reviewed by Miller and Miller (1976; see also Edds, 1973). Liver carcinomas have been observed in rats, ducks, rainbow trout, ferrets, and, to a limited extent, in mice, guinea pigs, and sheep. There are considerable differences in resistance to aflatoxin among species, with mouse, monkey, and probably man being quite resistant compared with the rat, fowl, and fish. Increased incidence of liver carcinomas has been reported in people in some parts of the world where the intake of aflatoxin B1 is very high (Pollock, 1979). The risk to the human population in the technologically advanced countries, however, is considered low owing to governmental regulatory agencies and industry that monitor human food and animal feed to prevent aflatoxin contamination. It should not present a problem to us if we utilize food in United States commerce.

Saccharin   Saccharin is not a potent carcinogen, but it is of great current concern in our country to many elderly people who consume considerable saccharin. The National Academy of Sciences issued a report on saccharin in 1978 in which they concluded that it is a weak bladder carcinogen in male rats. Consistent effects, however, were observed only in male rats fed saccharin diets during two consecutive generations.

Unlike most chemical carcinogens, saccharin is eliminated from the body essentially unchanged. After a careful study, Sweatman and Renwick (1979) concluded that saccharin is unusual in that its carcinogenic effects are due to the unmetabolized parent compound, and the mechanism involved in carcinogenesis remains undefined. Some workers suggest that saccharin has a promoter effect, that is, it may promote tumor formation in a tissue in which cells have been exposed to a carcinogen that has induced a tumor.

At our present stage of knowledge based on many decades of saccharin consumption, it seems reasonable to suggest that for the normal elderly person, moderate intake of saccharin-containing compounds will probably have little impact on health. We should not panic and rush to eliminate every substance found to cause cancer in laboratory animals until we have examined the study closely and carefully evaluated the alternatives. Recent incidence and mortality data on cancer suggest that the role of diet and food additives in carcinogenesis are exaggerated (Devesa and Silverman, 1978; Miller, personal communication, 1979).

ASSESSMENT OF RISK FROM CHEMICALS

To understand the significance of chemicals in our environment, especially at low levels, it is helpful to examine dose response curves used to evaluate risk at low levels of exposure. (Figure 14) The dose effect relationships are often expressed by two types of curves, a linear one that reflects an increasing effect that is proportional to dose, and a sigmoid one that reflects the fact that low doses may be less effective than an intermediate range of doses. Most of my scientific career has been directed at developing such dose response curves for various agents. For most agents, physical or chemical, we do not know the effects of very low doses on animals. At the intermediate and high range, enough animals can be economically used to obtain adequate information to plot effects. For illustrative purposes, one might look at solar radiation and sunburn. There are short exposures to the sun in which no redness of the skin is observed; but with higher doses redness

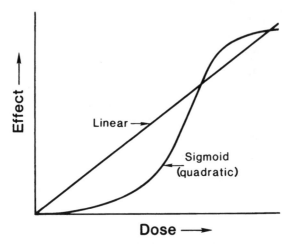

Figure 14. Dose effect curves showing linear and sig-
moidal response.

increases somewhat proportionally to the intensity of the
sun's rays and the time of exposure. The same might be said
of wind. A linear dose response curve on wind effects would
be as follows: In a given city with a 150-mile-an-hour wind
let us say 150 people would die, and if a 100-mile-an-hour
wind occurred, 100 people would die, and if a 50-mile-an-
hour wind occurred, 50 people would die. If this linear plot
were extended to zero wind speed, one would expect that
with a 5-mile-an-hour wind, 5 people would die and with a
1-mile-an-hour wind, 1 person would die. We can see in this
case that linearity extrapolated from dose effects obtained at
high exposure levels does not apply to low dose.

Similar situations occur with many agents, including the
chemicals discussed herein. Also important is that with lower
doses of certain chemicals or physical agents, not only is the
effect less, if perceptible, but the latency is also longer. It
may take a much longer time for the effect to be manifest,
that is, exposure at midlife may not be evident until very late
in life. With some agents, the latency may extend beyond a
normal life span. Another observation is that the steeper the

line on the linear curve, the more hazardous or dangerous the agent. In the older literature on toxicology we often dealt with the concepts of threshold; that is, for low levels of exposure there was no effect observed; the no-effect portion of the dose effect curve was followed by a curve of rapidly rising risks. A combination of these two curves is the low dose linear effect plus a higher dose (quadratic) curve. Most data today indicate that a quadratic model of dose effect is most applicable. In some cases, a low dose may be beneficial for some agents even though at high doses injury occurs. Unfortunately, with our present state of knowledge, for many agents for regulatory purposes and in determining safe limits most agencies use the linear curve. But determining risk for many agents using linear extrapolation may be unrealistic, expensive, and misleading (see Howard and Antilla, 1979).

Diet and Disease

FIBER

Changes in lifestyle and diet can reduce cancer incidence and mortality. The incidence of many cancers has fallen in this decade, but considerable epidemiological evidence indicates that dietary constituents may be significantly involved in the pathogenesis of several types of human and animal cancers. Both overnutrition and nutritional deficiencies have been implicated in an assortment of tumors, including those of the breast, colon, endometrium, kidney, ovary, pancreas, prostate, cervix, stomach, and thyroid.

Deaths from colon carcinoma are only exceeded by those due to carcinoma of the lung (which can be reduced by eliminating cigarette smoking). Colon cancer is a disease of the elderly; its increased incidence is very sharp beyond the age of forty. The disease appears to be at least partially diet-related, as are diverticulosis and gallstones. It is a disease that is strongly related to the lifestyle in Western Europe and the United States, as contrasted to that of residents in the developing countries. In emigrants from countries in which there is a low incidence of this disease, we find that within ten years of residency in the United States, the incidence approaches that of the native-born population of the United States (Haenszel, 1961). Extensive epidemiological studies of colon cancer rates have shown a remarkable correlation with dietary intake, especially of fat and high protein. Recently Enig and co-workers (1979) reported no correlation between animal protein and fat and colon cancer; they suggested transfatty acid intake may be implicated. Almy (1976) proposed that if a carcinogen in the colon is truly operative, a diet of sugars and refined cereals will contribute to a longer transit time of food in the colon, resulting in a higher concentration of any carcinogen to the epithelial surfaces. Bile acids and bile salts may be transformed by common bacteria in the human colon to carcinogens (Hill et al., 1971, 1975). It has been suggested that the interaction of bacteria and bile salts and the carcinogens produced in the intestines can be modified with the presence of dietary fiber. The evidence is such that little can be lost, and much possibly gained, by consuming more fiber, present in an assortment of fruits and vegetables.

Although fiber has received much attention in recent times, its benefits were heralded many years ago. In much of the Western world over the last 150 years, a remarkable decline has occurred in intake of crude vegetable fiber, although it was proposed about 140 years ago that people with diets lacking roughage were courting disaster (Graham, 1837). Recently we have come to recognize that certain gastrointestinal conditions of high prevalence in our society may be attributed to a deficiency of dietary fiber. Diseases implicated by this deficiency are chronic constipation, diverticulosis in the colon (along with colon carcinoma), gallbladder stones (cholelithiasis), hernias, hemorrhoids, and appendicitis. Lack of dietary fiber may also contribute to increased incidence of cardiovascular disease and diabetes. Graham noted that livestock could not be as healthy without the bulk of grain. He stated that whole grain would not only relieve constipation, but may correct diarrhea. Only recently, we have come to realize from the work of Burkitt et al. (1972) that dietary fiber could modify intestinal transit time (see Walker, 1975).

Hippocrates, 460-359 B.C., recognized the laxative effect of unbolted flour. The process of bolting involved sifting finely ground cereal and was developed by the early Egyptians. The Roman soldiers, who were at one time the most ingenious fighting force in the world, ate only bread made from coarse wheat flour, and the Spartans ate only very coarse bread from wheat to preserve their strength (Robinson, 1977).

Fiber is a complex substance that includes cellulose and hemicellulose, cutin, gum, lignin, mucin, pectin, waxes, and cell wall bound proteins. These substances may resist animal digestive enzymes but may undergo bacterial breakdown and fermentation in the colon ánd be absorbed (Holloway et al., 1978). Obviously, different fibers vary in their properties and in their effect on animals and people, depending on their source and preparation (Hegsted, 1977). In any case, if groups of animals are fed varying amounts of fiber, those fed the least amount develop more intestinal tumors. Binding or dilution of bile salts and fat degradation products by fiber also may explain their possible effectiveness (Upton, personal communication, 1979).

FAT

Dietary fat may have a promotional effect on cancer development and/or act as a solvent to enhance the effect of other carcinogens. Fats may also change the metabolism of certain tissues, possibly affecting hormonal effects on tissue growth. Other possibilities for carcinogenic action of fats may be their effect on structure and function of membranes, immunocompetence, and the DNA repair potential of the cell (Hopkins and West, 1976). Because of the widespread current concern about fats, an overview seems appropriate.

Although a great deal of research has been performed on fat intake, my "eighth law" is appropriately applied: The trouble ain't that people don't know anything; most of what they know ain't true. The literature on fat intake is fraught with controversy and misinformation (Enig et al., 1978; Applewhite, 1979; Bailar, 1979; Meyer, 1979; Enig et al., 1979).

Since misunderstanding exists regarding the classification
of lipids and fats, a brief discussion is warranted. Lipids are a
complex group of related compounds and include fats, oils,
waxes, and other compounds. Many fatty acids that derive
from fats are required in our diet. Those in natural fats usually
consist of an even number of carbon atoms and are what we
refer to as simple straight-chain fatty acids. The chain may be
saturated, that is, contain no double bonds, or be unsaturated,
containing one or more double bonds; if it contains two or
more double bonds it is called polyunsaturated fatty acid
(PUFA). The simplest and best known saturated fatty acid is
acetic ($CH_3 COOH$) acid and is common in the rumen of cattle. Among the most common in animal and plant fats are
palmitic ($C_{15} H_{33}$, COOH) and stearic acid ($C_{17} H_{35} COOH$).
A common polyunstaurated fatty acid and an essential one is
linoleic acid, found in seed oils like corn, cottonseed, peanut,
and soybeans. Often people use the terms "saturated" as syn-
onymous with animal fat, and "unsaturated" with vegetable-
derived fat; this is incorrect because polyunsaturates occur in
animal fat, and saturated fats occur in vegetable-derived fats
and oils. In fact, oils rich in polyunsaturated fatty acids are
usually hydrogenated, that is, the double bonds are filled in
with hydrogen to make them more stable and protect them
against heat damage. The result is a change in the normal *cis*
form of the fatty acid to a *trans* form that acts more like a
saturated fatty acid. There is great concern regarding transfatty acids today because their safety has been brought into
question. Our common food items like margarine, shortenings,
and dairy creamer substitutes may contain 15% to over 60%
transfatty acid. This subject is discussed more fully later.

   The consumption of animal fat as a source of dietary fat in
the United States has decreased over the last 70 years. At the
same time, the consumption of vegetable fat has increased almost threefold (Rizek et al., 1974; Gortner, 1975; Preston,
personal communication, 1979). The percentage of animal
fat in these and other references (in grams consumed per capita per day) was 83% of total fat intake; this has fallen to 62%

of the fat in the diet. An increase in total fat intake from 1909 until the 1970s was principally due to increases in unsaturated fat rather than saturated fat (from 21 g to 59 g per person per day.)

Some workers have reported that beef was the major source of saturated fat for the adult in the United States (Wynder and Reddy, 1975). The data I found (Rizek et al., 1974) indicated that saturated fat from vegetable fat in 1965 was greater than that from beef (9.8 g versus 9.2 g). In fact, there appears to have been more saturated fat in the diet from vegetable fat than from beef since 1929. It is also of some consequence that the various vegetable oils and margarine vary in their saturation. Soybean and corn oil contain approximately 10% saturated fatty acids prior to refining. However, after processing they contain approximately 15% to 25% saturated fatty acids depending on whether they are marketed as margarine, oil, or shortening. Cottonseed oil is 25% saturated before processing, while coconut oil is 85% saturated before processing (see also Enig et al., 1978).

Epidemiological data are enlightening but also confusing relative to the incidence of breast and colon cancer and dietary fat intake. It is interesting to note that the Greek population has less than one-fourth the incidence of breast cancer compared with Israel, but has about the same total dietary fat intake. Spain has about one-third the breast cancer mortality of France and Italy, but the total dietary fat intake in Spain is slightly greater than in these other two countries. Relative to high animal fat intake, Puerto Rico has an animal fat intake of 106 grams but a very low rate of colon and breast cancer. In Puerto Rico, the animal fat represents about 88% of the total fat, whereas in the United States only 65% of the fat is animal fat, yet the breast and colon cancer rates in Puerto Rico are only about one-third those of the United States. Other interesting data come from the Netherlands and Finland, where the daily intake per capita of animal fat is about 100 grams. Breast and colon cancer rates in the Netherlands are almost twice those observed in Finland, yet the animal fat intake in the Netherlands is only 65% of the total fat, and in Finland it represents 88%. Intake of vegetable fat per day is four times greater in the Netherlands than in Finland (53 g as compared with 13 g). Data from American Indians in the Southwest is also interesting. They are known to have a high animal fat intake but very low breast cancer rates. In a study of the different social and economic classes in Columbia, it was found that the higher income economic classes had a fourfold excess risk for colon cancer, while they consumed less animal fat than the lower economic classes (Enig et al., 1978).

It is interesting to note that the Seventh Day Adventists have a lower colon cancer rate than the general population. The Seventh Day Adventist physicians have a significantly higher rate of colon cancer, however, than non-Seventh Day Adventist physicians. It appears inconceivable that the Seventh Day Adventist physicians eat more animal fat and beef than non-Seventh Day Adventist physicians. Obviously, other factors are involved. When considering the hazards of fat intake, one must consider all sources of fat.

The major change in the intake of fat in the United States in this century has been an increase in the consumption of partially hydrogenated vegetable fats, including margarines, vegetable shortenings, and oils. The critical issue in this regard may be that they contain significant quantities of altered, unsaturated fatty acids containing trans double bonds in place of the natural cis double bonds. Trans fatty acids differ from the naturally occurring cis form in the manner in which they are incorporated into triglycerides and phospholipids. Trans fatty acid isomers are present in levels of up to 17% in commercial vegetable oils, over 60% in some margarines (Ottenstein, 1976), and 58% in vegetable shortenings. Calculations indicate that the trans fatty acid content of the diets in 1910 was only about 4.4 grams, but this almost tripled by the 1970s. Recently, Beare-Rogers and associates (1979) expressed concern that in analysis of 50 brands of margarines, high concentrations of trans fatty acids tended to be associated with low linoleic acid (a vital fatty acid). It has also been noted that some human tissues are reported to contain up to 14% trans fatty acids (Enig et al., 1978; Kummerow et al., 1977 and others).

Correlations noted by Enig suggested that vegetable fats, but not animal fats, were highly correlated with the increase in cancer rates. This is consistent with the data of Tannenbaum in 1942 when he suggested a possible role for dietary fat in the causation of cancer in laboratory animals. He used hydrogenated cottonseed oil and soybean oil. Carroll (1975) and Carroll and Khor (1971) have further examined this possibility, using more refined oils that reportedly contain 17% trans fatty acids if partially hydrogenated (see also Dutton, 1974).

Several animal studies have indicated that the type of dietary fat consumed rather than the caloric content of the diet affects the incidence of spontaneously occurring or induced tumors. Rogers and Newberne (1975) observed fewer tumors in the colon of laboratory animals on a diet of 28% beef fat than in controls fed 15% corn oil.

Several other investigators have demonstrated that increased amounts of dietary fat, in particular polyunsaturated fat, increase the incidence of some spontaneous and induced tumors. Tannenbaum reported a higher incidence and shorter latent period of spontaneous mammary tumors in mice fed a high fat diet versus those on a low fat diet. The work of Carroll's group has shown that the incidence of mammary tumors induced by 7,12-dimethylbenz (a) anthracene (DMBA) is increased by feeding rats a high fat diet containing polyunsaturated fat rather than a low fat diet or a high fat diet containing saturated fat (Carroll and Khor, 1971). Carroll and Khor reported that there tended to be more tumors per rat when unsaturated fats were fed, and this was reflected in a trend towards higher tumor yields with increased unsaturation of the diets. Obviously, more work needs to be done. Suffice it to say our diet should not contain over about 25-30% fat and the amount of transfatty acid consumed should be restricted until its long-term safety is determined. In this regard, a concerted effort should be made to require testing of its safety immediately and also require that its content in all fats and oils be indicated clearly on the label. This is a serious omission in today's labeling (M. Hegsted, personal communication, 1979; Johnson, personal communication, 1979).

ALCOHOL

Although no conclusive proof exists that alcohol alone causes cancer, a good deal of evidence suggests that high alcohol consumption in combination with smoking and dietary deficiencies may cause increased cancer incidence. Alcohol is an irritant of the lining cells of the throat, esophagus, and stomach, and when combined with chemical and physical irritants, leads to increased incidence of cancer in the mouth, larynx, throat, and esophagus.

VITAMINS AND MINERALS

Certain vitamins are thought to have anticarcinogenic properties. Vitamin A has been proposed as a preventive agent for some common epithelial cancers. But the data for people is tenuous, and vitamin A is known to be toxic in high amounts. A riboflavin deficiency increased the production of liver tumors in rats fed a carcinogen, while a riboflavin-containing coenzyme was essential for destruction of the carcinogen (Miller and Miller, 1953). Vitamin C is known to interact with ingested nitrites and nitrates and may thereby have anticarcinogenic effects by inhibiting nitrosamine formation. Limited studies in people have suggested that vitamin C has caused regression of rectal polyps. Dietary choline was found to inhibit the induction of tumors in rats fed an aflatoxin containing diet (Newberne, 1965). Certain minerals including zinc, selenium, iron, and magnesium have been proposed as anticarcinogens, but their efficacy is not proved. Unfortunately, in hopes of curing cancer or other conditions, people have consumed these substances in amounts high enough to cause toxicity (Theologides, personal communication, 1979).

Restricting food intake has affected tumor incidence in some studies. Before I was born — in fact, about 65 years ago,

Peyton Rous (1911) noted that by restricting food intake in mice, the development of mammary tumor transplants and metastases was delayed. It wasn't until 30 and 40 years later that related findings were described in rats and people where food restriction was shown to diminish the incidence of both carcinogen-induced and spontaneous tumors (Rusch, 1944; Tannenbaum and Silverstone, 1953). Boutwell (1964, 1974) found that animals whose food intake was severely restricted manifested activated pituitary and adrenal glands and increased adrenal cortical hormone levels.

Although of limited applicability, it appears that moderate stress through caloric restriction (Tannenbaum and Silverstone, 1953) and probably exercise may protect people against cancer formation. Studies in people, however, are limited, and the present state of knowledge regarding restricting dietary intake has little application to elderly people.

Osteoporosis and Periodontal Disease

Osteoporosis, a metabolic bone disease characterized by substantial reduction in total bone mass, is another condition that may be affected by vitamins and minerals. The disease affects approximately 30% or more of the women over 55 and men over 60 years, and is four times as prevalent in women. About 12 million people in the United States are afflicted with this disease. Some estimate up to 50% of postmenopausal women in the United States have this disease (Smith and Rizek, 1966). Although the cause is not known, patients with osteoporosis often consume insufficient protein, have a low caloric intake, and some may have a lifelong aversion to dairy foods and hence low calcium and vitamin D intake (Urist, 1973a, b; see also Barzel, 1970, 1978). Dietary deficiencies are implicated in the rat and some other animals, but may be less important in people (Gordan & Vaughan, 1976; Gordan, personal communication, 1979). Gordan believes low estrogen levels are critical factors in postmenopausal women who develop osteoporosis. Some workers believe intestinal malabsorption and reduced kidney function may also contribute (Jee, personal communication, 1979; Posner, 1979). The disease in people is characterized by increased susceptibility to vertebral and other fractures, backache and other pain, vertebral deformities, and progressive loss of height.

Few satisfactory animal models exist for osteoporosis in postmenopausal women. Although the ovariectomized rat will manifest an osteoporosis, it is not considered a suitable model for people (Jee, personal communication, 1979). Work on chickens with cage layer osteoporosis has been instructive (Urist, 1960). Very recent work on female pigtail macaques indicate they are similar to aging females (Bowden, et al., 1979; see also Lei and Yong, 1979). Spencer has written about swine model for lactational osteoporosis (1979).

Of related interest and of great concern for the elderly is periodontal disease, which causes the loss of teeth in approximately 35 million people in this country (most of whom are elderly). Periodontitis may be a concomitant expression of osteoporosis (Lutwak et al., 1971; Weg, 1978). Studies to test the hypothesis that periodontal disease represents a type of osteoporosis suggested that the strength of supporting bone (for example, resulting from Ca supplementation) may be important in preventing the development of periodontitis.

Recommendations for the elderly with these "bone diseases" include small doses of sex hormone, for example, conjugated estrogen, which may arrest the disease and reduce the number of fractures (Urist, 1973b). Gordan recommends 0.3 mg premarin per day (Gordan, personal communication, 1979). For the diet, it seems prudent in view of conflicting data and variability among individuals that those approaching 60 consume at least 1 g calcium daily and adequate amounts of vitamin C and D. Relative to vitamin D, a dose of 1,000 I.U./day is generally sufficient unless a malabsorption condition exists. Larger doses of vitamin D are toxic and can cause harmful calcification of arterial walls and kidneys. Calcium intake and absorption appear to fall with age, and phosphorus intake usually remains high, thus changing the Ca:P ratio from a desirable 2:1 to 1:4. At this stage of our knowledge, fluorine supplementation is not recommended. Exercise is strongly recommended and appears to be important (Urist, 1971a, b, 1973a, b).

Mental Disorders

Recently I was reviewing an edition of the magazine *Nature* and the first title that caught my eye was "Dementia: an approaching epidemic," by my one-time professor at the University of Washington School of Medicine, Fred Plum (1979). Dr. Plum stated that: "Dementia is overwhelmingly a problem of man's declining years and in the Western world both the percentage and actual numbers of the susceptible population are increasing at an alarming rate." He went on to state the estimated annual cost for caring for chronic dementia patients is 12 billion dollars (which is almost 5 times the present total budget of the National Institutes of Health). In 50 years, it is projected to be 30 billion dollars annually in present dollar value. As impressive as this problem is to the taxpayer, it is even more devastating to the elderly person and his or her family. Irene Mortenson Burnside, in a very thoughtful and sensitive presentation on mental health, recalled a session with elderly people regarding their greatest concerns (Burnside, 1975a, b). Without hesitation, they cited loneliness, depression, brain damage, and the meaninglessness of their lives. It appears that some of these conditions are amenable to amelioration nutritionally or by other reasonable means.

The chronic brain syndrome denotes all of the organic mental deteriorations that occur in the elderly (Shelanski, 1975). The term "senile dementia" is sometimes used for an assortment of diseases including Alzheimer's Disease, Pick's Disease, cerebral vascular insufficiencies, and sometimes Creutzfeldt-Jakob Disease and tardive dyskinesia. Some regard these entities as aging phenomena and not diseases, characterized by a slow onset with subtle manifestations. One sees increased irritability, loss of initiative, procrastination, confusion, memory loss, and difficulty in adaptation to new environmental situations or environmental stresses. The symptoms may not become noticeable until a person faces a change in his or her situation, such as retirement. Anxiety increases and more serious symptoms may result.

Alzheimer's senile dementia causes more functional disability in the elderly than all other chronic brain diseases listed above (Plum, 1979). This disease was well summarized in a recent NIH-sponsored workshop. Alzheimer's Disease may have a genetic component; anatomical changes indicate an acceleration of the normal aging process that may be independent of cardiovascular disease. Some recent work indicates that a specific neurochemical system may be involved that may respond to pharmacotherapy (Kendall, 1979). But we must devote more research monies to understanding cell systems that transact functions of memory, learning, and judgment.

In 1976, Wurtman observed that acetylcholine (a neurotransmitter) synthesis increased in rat brains when the animals were fed large amounts of choline. This was an exciting development, for it changed the thinking of many relative to the activity of neurons in response to fluctuations in the diet. Wurtman and associates had reported that the rate that the brain synthesizes neurotransmitters changes in accordance with the amounts of the precursors for these transmitters in the blood (see Davies, 1978). Within a few months after Wurtman and associates reported their work on rats, Davis and associates at Stanford gave large doses of choline to a patient that suffered from tardive dyskinesia, and they reported an improvement (see Kolata, 1979). Their report was followed by several others in a very short time. This, of course, was welcome news, since up to half of the patients in many state mental hospitals suffer from this very disturbing disease that manifests itself by varying disfigurements of the face, including involuntary twitches of facial muscles, rolling tongue, lip smacking, lip puckering, and rapid eye blinking.

Choline is not a universal cure, but it has certainly improved the condition in many people, especially those who were on antipsychotic drugs that depress acetycholine. If the patients have been too long on an antipsychotic drug or are suffering from a long-term senile condition, there may be no response. Lecithin, rather than choline, is probably the best source of this drug, since choline itself is broken down by bacteria in the alimentary tract and, as a result, patients receiving the drug have a very fishy smell. This does not happen when lecithin is given, for it appears to be absorbed by the intestinal mucosa and is not degraded by bacteria. One should strive to obtain pure lecithin, which will be more readily available soon.

Other conditions, such as Alzheimer's Disease, are also being studied in relationship to choline. In the case of mania, choline may be used with lithium, which is a fairly toxic material. It has been observed that when rats were given lithium, the effectiveness of the dietary choline in increasing brain acetylcholine was enhanced.

As a result of the work with choline, other investigations have been initiated using dietary elements, such as the amino acids tryptophan and tyrosine, which are precursors for the catecholamine transmitters. Investigators propose that these substances might be useful in the treatment of depression.

One of our failings in geriatric medicine, whether we deal with people or pets, is that whenever an ailing aged patient is presented we are too prone to chalk everything up to inevitable, age-related changes. Many aging phenomena can be readily treated and/or alleviated.

Loneliness is another psychological disorder of concern to the elderly, often occurring with the loss of relationships and the inability to find new relationships. This emotional problem is even more important than those discussed earlier in this chapter. I am sure Wesley Spink, whom we honor with these lectures, and Robert Butler, director of the National Council of Aging, who wrote the foreword to this volume, both would agree that depression, meaninglessness, and rejection by society, the feelings associated with the loneliness that plagues so many elderly, are the worst things that can happen to a person or a sentient animal. Most people think of human closeness as the only antidote for loneliness (Burnside, 1976a, b). As discussed in Chapter 4, companion animals have proved to be not only a good antidote for loneliness, but also for depression and a feeling of meaninglessness. Animals serve as social integrators, introducing the owners to new situations and people, and give them something to live for—responsibility for a dependent and lovable life (Corson and Corson, 1979; Levinson, 1969b; Walster, 1979).

The usual dog, for example, is exceedingly friendly to its master or mistress and provides a warm welcome whether the absence is a three-minute visit to the basement or a week-long trip. Obviously, most dogs have unqualified positive regard for the owner, no matter what his or her appearance, condition, or lot in life. The results in many cases have been phenomenal; yet this modestly priced therapy is little recognized by the health science profession. In fact, in an otherwise useful and comprehensive text on the clinical aspects of aging, no mention is made of the usefulness of animals for helping old people (see Reichel, 1978).

Educational Considerations in Geriatric Medicine

We in clinical veterinary medicine have several advantages over the physician in human medicine in that our professional life span usually exceeds that of most of our patients. Also, our patients follow instructions better because the owners, although they may not follow recommendations from their own physicians for themselves, are highly motivated to look after their animals. In addition, we more readily recognize the uniqueness of each patient because of the striking differences in breeds and species. For example, a two-pound Manchester and a 150-pound Irish Wolfhound are obviously different, even though they may be the same age and have the same owner. Since we become familiar with family situations and often with the entire life span of a cat or a dog, we are able to administer to the animal in a family situation with a better knowledge of its history.

As an animal patient ages, we can readily introduce a young animal as a helpful partner. After a short period of adjustment, the young pet usually helps the physical and psychological well-being of the older pet and assists the client in adjustment when the older anmal dies or is euthanized.

In clinical veterinary medicine, we do not have, as far as I know, departments of geriatric medicine (see Stout, 1979; Williamson, 1979). But we realize the importance of integrating all our knowledge in treating the aging animal. In human medicine, we also need a broad knowledge of the entire field of medicine to deal effectively with the elderly. In this regard, William Hazzard (1979) wisely said:

In the aged patient in whom multi-system, multi-disease, multi-problem presentation is the rule rather than the exception, such judgment, coupled with a compassionate appreciation of the contribution of the social and physical environment to disability and its conquest or endurance is the essence of good, medical practice.

He went on to say that geriatrics may, in fact, be the last haven of the general physician because of the complex and subtle judgments required when multiple problems may blur diagnostic borders and may even inhibit aggressive diagnosis and treatment.

Having said this, I do not discount the great need for divisions or programs in gerontology and geriatric medicine. We need specialists in chronic disease and extended care. Incentives and encouragement must be offered for this important branch of knowledge in view of the ignorance in this area and the increasing populations that will require an expanded data bank and technology. As one who has helped many of the elderly in retirement and convalescent homes, I believe there is a lack of well-trained physicians in the area of chronic disease and long-term care. We lack knowledge and understanding of the older patient and the older client and do not fully realize the problems of the elderly (see Beeson, 1979; Solon, 1978).

Dr. Butler, now the director of the National Aging Institute, recalled his days as a medical student at Columbia University, where he heard a lot of discussion about "crocks" among young interns, as well as among attending physicians and residents. The name "crock" was often used to refer to an undesirable patient beyond middle age who had a multiplicity of complaints. Often they were stroke victims. He would also hear people describing older persons as having "serum porcelain levels"; this was an inside joke, probably elaborating on the word crock. To say that an old person was "super tentorial" meant that his illness was all in his mind. He heard many other terms that were derogatory such as "old fogie," "snag," "rounder," "shopper," "floater," "geezer" and "constitutionally inadequate." Dr. Butler recalled, too, the group clinic that was part of the training in the third year to give students the opportunity to see real illness, that is, organic illness unencumbered by emotional problems. In this service, patients were carefully screened, and yet he and others estimated that up to 50% had psychological problems that were often a major component of their illness, but were ignored. It was just such an experience that interested Dr. Butler in psychiatry.

He also noted an overemphasis on teaching and research rather than on decent service and humane treatment. He went on to point out that although 20 years have passed since his medical training, the attitudes have not changed appreciably in the areas in which he travels. In his studies at the University of California, he interviewed medical students there, and concluded that at no point in their medical education are students exposed to any systematic consideration of the nature of old people and their medical and social problems. As a result, the students retain the sum of society's misconceptions about old people and are therefore likely to discriminate against them in medical practice (Butler, 1975; see Bevan, 1972; Birenbaum et al., 1979).

We must emphasize in the medical curriculum the importance of the reverence for life, including life of the elderly.

In this regard, I'm reminded of C. S. Lewis' (1946) words:

It is a serious thing to live in a society of possible gods and goddesses, to remember that the dullest and most uninteresting person you talk to may one day be a creature which, if you saw it now, you would be strongly tempted to worship, or else a horror and a corruption such as you now meet, if at all, only in a nightmare. All day long we are, in some degree, helping each other to one or other of these destinations.

Part of the reverence for life for all of us in the health professions includes knowing how to handle death and grief. This includes grief manifested by a patient for loss of family members or a much-loved companion animal. We will not be able to handle this if we have not faced the inevitability of our own death and experienced the insight and compassion this confirmation gives us in dealing with the life around us.

CHAPTER 4

THE CONTRIBUTIONS
OF COMPANION ANIMALS
TO HUMAN WELL-BEING

The heart is hard in nature, and unfit
For human fellowship, as being void
Of sympathy, and therefore dead alike
To love and friendship, that is not pleased
With the sight of animals enjoying life,
Nor feels their happiness augment his own.
(William Cowper, 1785)

Many older people, some for the first time in their lives, have discovered that companion animals satisfy some of their greatest needs, restore order to their lives, and enable them to grasp more securely the world of reality, the world of caring, concern, sacrifice, and intense emotional relationships. If older people withdraw from active participation in human affairs, the nonhuman environment becomes increasingly important. At this time in their lives, the elderly can gain much from companion animals. Animals can provide a boundless measure of acceptance, adoration, attention, forgiveness, and unconditional love. Animals also contribute to their owners' concept of self-worth and sense of being needed. The animal they care for loves them in return; in fact, it will often sacrifice its life for them. This is no small matter.

The potential for good to many varieties and conditions of people exists in innumerable ways through companion animals. But, even though companion animals have been with us for thousands of years, few data exist on the measurable

116

therapeutic benefits of the people-pet bond. However, a review of the history of pet-facilitated therapy provides valuable insight into the positive aspects and potential.

Landmarks in the Use of Animals in Therapy

In most publications, the York Retreat is cited as the first instance of therapy involving animals. In 1792 this unique retreat was founded by the Society of Friends. York Retreat was the brain child of William Tuke, a Quaker tea and coffee merchant who started the Retreat at a time when lunatic hospitals and asylums often treated their patients very badly. It was neither a hospital nor a private asylum, but was financed and organized on a nonprofit basis by a restricted membership. The retreat employed a form of treatment based on "Christianity and common sense" (Jones, 1955).

York Retreat was, of necessity, an experiment, because reform was impossible until some system of treatment other than that operational in the lunatic hospitals and asylums had been tried and found successful. An open-minded physician was engaged who believed that "moral methods" of treatment were preferable to those involving restraint and harsh drugs. The Tuke family felt that many patients would be rational and could be controlled if they were not aggravated by cruelty, harsh methods of restraint, and hostility. Accordingly, the patients at York Retreat were never punished for failure to control their behavior. Instead, kindness and understanding were extended to them in order to foster self-control by a show of trust. At regular tea parties, the patients were encouraged to wear their very best clothes instead of the "institutional garb" of most asylums.

Most significantly, each of the court areas at the Retreat contained a number of small animals, including rabbits and poultry, so that the patients might learn self-control by caring for creatures dependent on them. The patients busily cared for the animals, helped in the garden, and knitted and sewed. They could use writing materials, read books from a carefully chosen library for patients, and attend religious services. The patients were made to feel accepted rather than barred from participation in normal human activity or cut off from the outside world. The staff stressed curative and soothing effects of warm baths for the patients, and also an abundant diet of meat, bread, and good porter (a heavy, ale-like beer). The Tuke family felt this diet was a far more effective policy than semistarvation, and they regarded porter as successful as opium in inducing sound sleep, while being less detrimental to the body.

Seventy-five years later, in 1867, Bethel in Bielefeld, Germany, was founded and animals were an integral part of the enterprise. It began modestly as a home for epileptics (Funke and Hocke, personal communication, 1977) but is now an extensive center of healing for disadvantaged people, with over 5,000 patients and more than 5,000 staff members. When I visited Bethel in 1977, I noted that the complex seemed to be patterned somewhat after the York Retreat described above (Bustad, 1978b). Birds, cats, dogs, and horses are evident in many of the residences and work sites, in addition to farm animals and a wild game park. I asked my host how long pets had been utilized with their patients. He said they only recently began using horses, but he thought they had kept other pets since the very early years. They realize that using pets to help people is natural, just common sense, and accept it as an appropriate and reasonable way of life. However, they have not recorded observations on the impact of animals on patients or developed studies to determine quantitatively the animals' worthiness and benefits. They just know animals are helpful (Hocke, personal communication, 1977).

The first recorded use of animals in therapy in the United States occurred in the 1940s at the Pawling Army Air Force Convalescent Hospital in Pawling, New York. The Pawling Center received Air Force personnel from every theater of operations and from every segment of the globe during World War II. The patients, convalescing from injuries or recovering from the effects of operational fatigue, needed a regime of restful activity rather than continued medical treatment. An academic program was designed to keep their minds active and, at the same time, give them surcease from war and its activities. The patients were encouraged to work at the Center's farm with hogs, cattle, horses, and poultry. They also benefited from the healing powers of snakes, frogs, turtles, and other living creatures of the field and forest, along with the fields and forests themselves (Menning, personal communication, 1979).

A Backyard Exploration Group organized frog-jumping contests and turtle races. Members of the group captured the frogs from the Center's frog pond and entered their charges in the contest, which was held in a 12-foot circle. The competitive spirit made the contests very popular and, at the same time, gave the men a keen insight into the lives and habits of frogs.

After World War II, a more concerted effort was directed towards using companion animals in therapy. Dr. Boris Levinson discovered the great advantages of companion animals after a mother and her disturbed offspring arrived several hours early for an appointment. Since Dr. Levinson was not expecting patients, he had his dog, Jingles, with him in his office. This accidental meeting of Jingles and the child was the key to the eventual rehabilitation of the patient. Levinson launched a career of using companion animals in therapy and promoting their use in many rewarding situations. He also called for systematic studies of their effectiveness. His plea for rigorous research to establish boundaries and princi- ples was accompanied by the caution that we must learn how to select and train animals for special psychotherapeutic work (Levinson, 1961, 1966, 1968, 1969a, b, 1972, 1974).

Sam and Elizabeth Corson and their associates took up Levinson's charge at Ohio State University, where they were among the first to attempt systematically to evaluate pet-facilitated therapy (Corson, et al., 1975, 1977, 1979). They began with a colony of dogs housed in a psychiatric hospital, one floor below the day room of a psychiatric ward. Like Levinson, the Corsons entered this field of study through unexpected circumstances. One of the patients heard the dogs barking and wanted to visit them. The Corsons, after much thought, decided that using pets for patients who had failed to respond to so-called "standard" therapy (e.g., drugs and electroshock) was worth investigating. From a mixture of collies, beagles, cocker spaniels, and wire-haired terriers, they attempted to match the temperaments of the dogs with the needs of specific patients.

The results of the Corsons' experiments were exceedingly encouraging. Many psychotics who were bedridden and un-communicative were transformed and eventually discharged. The Corsons reasoned that the pets were effective in psycho-therapy because, to a withdrawn individual, the pets are un-demanding, uncritical friends who serve as loving links for those who have lost social skills and desires. Furthermore, the pets need their help; they need to be fed, bathed, and brushed. As the patients assumed these duties, the Corsons noted that the patients began taking better care of themselves.

Similar positive results were realized when the dogs were moved to the Castle Nursing Home in Millersburg, Ohio. The well-identified and categorized dogs were a very welcome ad-dition to the home for the elderly residents, many of whom were bedridden or in wheelchairs. These animals were effec-tive social matchmakers in that they aided the elderly resi-dents in relating to other residents and nursing home per-sonnel. The dogs helped to transform dependent, infantile, self-neglecting behavior into more responsible and self-re-liant action. Some patients took the dogs for walks and even ran with them, thereby increasing the physical activity and general well-being of both. Pups were especially help-ful to mentally retarded residents. One person nearly 80 years old had spoken very little for several decades, and what he said was difficult to understand. On seeing a dog he said, "You brought that dog." Then he asked if he could keep it (Figure 15). This brought him out of his shell, and he be-gan relating to the staff, tracing pictures of dogs, and then producing excellent free-hand drawings of dogs (Corson, per-

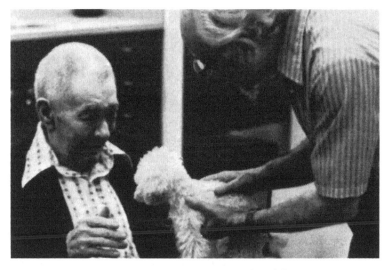

Figure 15. Sam Corson with Jed and dog.

sonal communication, 1979). He became a happier person and was more willing to relate to people (Corson and Corson, 1979).

The Corsons recorded progress of the patients after the introduction of dogs by a simple questionnaire that nurses completed. Videotapes were made of resident-pet-staff interactions. Such recordings made it possible to quantify temporal and verbal parameters of the patients' responses. The tapes also served as therapeutic feedback modalities for the residents.

In 1966, a rehabilitation center for handicapped people, Beitostolen, was established in a ski area in central Norway. The motivating force was Erling Stordahl, a blind musician, and his wife, who believed a new approach was needed for the handicapped. In addition to an active physical therapy and sports program, the center uses dogs and horses as an important component of the therapy regimen. Blind people learn how to ski and ride horses there. Because of the great success of this program, Norwegians associated with Beitostolen have purchased land in Minnesota near the Twin Cities as a gift to the United States, where they hope a similar rehabilitation center might be established (Krog, personal communication, 1971, 1978).

Benefits of Animals to Human Health

In the very recent past, two important studies by Friedmann (1979) and by Mugford and M'Comisky (1975) have provided valuable data on the specific benefits of animals to human health. We know that breakdown of the family, geographic and social mobility, neighborhood and institutional deterioration, and social isolation adversely affect the emotional and physical health of people. Our strongest evidence for this is in mortality statistics (Friedmann, 1979) that reveal that divorced, single, and widowed individuals have a higher age-specific death rate than do those who are married. If one could identify those who are happily married, the difference would probably be even greater. These same "disadvantaged" people also suffer a higher morbidity owing to an assortment of behavioral disorders and degenerative diseases. We know that among surviving mates, the death rate increases in the first two years of their grief, especially when one adds data for people under 65. This increase may, in great part, be caused by the depression and loneliness that result from the absence of companionship that provided positive behavioral and emotional effects. Even in dogs, I have observed the physical deterioration of an animal after the death of a close, long-term animal or human companion.

Friedmann (1979) recalled certain studies that indicated that lack of social support may be related to the incidence of coronary heart disease, but noted no one had definitively studied the relationship between social support and survival following coronary heart disease. Therefore, they undertook to gather basic data. In a two-year period, in a corporate study at the University of Pennsylvania and the University of Maryland, they studied all patients admitted to a large university hospital with a diagnosis of either angina pectoris or myocardial infarction. A total of 189 patients were interviewed,

Table 8. Relationship of Pet Ownership to One-Year Survival

Patients	No Pet	Pet	Total
Alive	28	50	78
Not Alive	11	3	14
Total	39	53	92

Chi Square = 8.9 p < 0.02 (Friedman, 1979).

and informed consent was obtained from all those who were involved in the study. In the initial interview, the investigators inventoried the social data and psychological mood status of each patient. Included in the social inventory was the socioeconomic status, social network, geographic mobility, and living situation. Pet ownership was one of the items included in the long list of information obtained. Only those 92 patients whose physiological data was complete, including electrocardiograms and enzyme analysis at time of discharge, were included in the study. One year after discharge, all of the patients were contacted. Table 8 lists the results.

It is obvious from Table 8 that significantly more pet owners than nonpet owners survived one year. Since owning a pet, especially a dog, requires some exertion on the part of the owner, it was possible that the pet owner actually exerted more physical effort, and this in itself might modify the survival rate. So, Friedmann and associates made a comparison between patients who had a pet other than a dog and patients who owned no pets. Ten persons had pets other than dogs, and none of these subjects died. Of the 39 subjects without pets, 11 had died. The relationship between pet ownership and survival remained significant, even when subjects owning dogs were eliminated from the analysis.

These workers also investigated the relationship between pet ownership and severity of cardiovascular disease. They found that pet ownership was correlated with survival but not with physiological severity. Thus, it appears that the relationship between survival and pet ownership is not dependent on the physiological state of the patient. Friedmann found that none of the other variables, such as the number of people that were talked to each day, the amount of daily contact with neighbors, the participation in community activities, or living alone or being married explained as much of the variance in survival as did pet ownership. She reported that pet ownership by itself is related to one-year survival of patients who were hospitalized for either angina pectoris or myocardial infarction. Her findings raise an interesting question: What is the source of the apparent influence of companion animals on survival: We have to admit we do not know.

Pets, of course, ameliorate loneliness and help fill the need for companionship. However, this explanation does not answer the question entirely, since survival did not appear to be greater among the married. The frequency of contacts with family and friends or the patients' involvement in social activities did not influence one-year survival, either. It appears that companion animals do not act only as substitutes for the beneficial effects of human contact, or affect only the lonely and isolated.

Perhaps the apparent effects of companion animals on survival may not be dependent on the pet at all, but be a result of differences in social condition or personality between those who choose to have pets and those who do not. The coronary prone behavior pattern type A is associated with the development of heart disease. Perhaps the patient's personality, and not pet ownership, determines survival. Friedmann and associates, however, found no difference in the measures of tension, anxiety, depression, confusion, vigor, or fatigue between those who did, and those who did not, own pets. (Investigation is needed on possible personality differences as related to pet ownership.)

We recognize that there are social differences between people who keep companion animals and people who do not. In the Friedmann study, the people with pets tended to be raised in a rural environment and live in their current living situations longer; they owned homes and lived with a family. The black subjects who had companion animals had higher incomes and were married as well. These factors would tend to favor survival. But the answer to why pet owners survived in greater percentages is elusive.

As indicated earlier, the "ancients" recognized that keeping animals contributed to the health of the owners. Many people seem to accept this belief without exploring the reason of pursuing it in a scientific way. Anecdotal information has multiplied recently relative to the benefits of keeping companion animals. We know that varied and interesting daily activities are reasonable social predictors of longevity (Youmans and Yarrow, 1971; Libow, 1963); pets require attention and regular duties every day for people who often have no other reason for scheduled activity. They also provide companionship and facilitate socializing with other people (Siegel, 1962; Levinson, 1969a, b; Mugford, 1979a, b). A Swedish study showed that over half of the owners' introductions and opportunities to communicate with people were pet initiated (Bath et al., 1976). Corson made similar observations with psychiatric patients and the staff of a hospital (Corson and Corson, 1979).

For old people, too often in the family and especially outside the family, attention and love are not common commodities. Companion animals may be a significant part and, in some cases, the only source of warmth, affection, love, and devotion for the elderly. Pets seem to negate some of the unfortunate health effects of the stresses of living. In many cases, pets give people a good reason or a need for living.

The importance of touch is often discounted but may, in part, explain the importance of contact comfort, especially to the male population. We know that the petting of a dog or a horse causes a profound change in the animal's cardiovascular response (Anderson and Garritt, 1966; Lynch and McCarthy, 1967, 1969; Lynch, et al., 1974; Katcher, 1979). We may be dealing with a direct physiological effect by active presence of the animal and petting. Work of Lacey et al. (1963) suggests that the pleasure of watching animals, whether birds, fish, or other companion animals, relaxes the observer (Benson et al., 1978). The same relaxation may be characteristic in the communication with animals without speech. Expecting a response from an animal may also be very salutary, as may the animal's response.

Earlier than the study by Friedmann and associates, Mugford and M'Comisky (1975) conducted an interesting quantitative study of the therapeutic role of animals for elderly people in East Yorkshire, England (near Hull). The subjects were 75- to 81-year-old pensioners living in an urban setting; they were relatively isolated due to immobility. The authors' stated objective was to "determine the feasibility of field experimentation into the effects of pets upon the social attitudes and mental and physical health of their owners."

Five groups of six members each were established:

* Groups 1 and 2 owned television sets
* Groups 3 and 4 did not
* Group 5 had an equal number of owners and nonowners of television sets.

All participants were interviewed by a male psychologist and a female social worker. At the time of the interview, a small gift was given to each person to establish a good rapport. All members of groups 1 and 3 were then given a budgerigar (a small Australian parrot usually called a budgie), and members of groups 2 and 4 were given begonias. Special emphasis was accorded to television ownership, since television watching might diminish the effectiveness of a budgie companion.

The questionnaire consisted of 30 items in three sections. The first section explored attitudes toward other people. The second section asked how the members regarded themselves relative to their physical and psychological well-being and their attitude toward their environment. The third section concentrated on demographic data, including age and details of family. During the study period of five months, all of the members of each group were visited by the social worker each month. On the fifth month, the questionnaire was again administered, to determine any change in attitudes. Membership in the groups suffered a 40% attrition during the four months. Factors influencing this study included death of a relative or a friend of the subject, chronic or sudden illness, change in the situation of the subject, and friends visiting at the time of the interview.

Evaluation showed an overall positive effect of the pets. All 12 budgie recipients insisted on making their own arrangements for the food and other material that the budgies required. Although the experiment ceased after five months, the people still owned their budgies and were taking good care of them 18 months later. Soon after receiving them, all 12 recipients gave the budgies endearing names. All except one of the male subjects trained the birds to leave the cage, while all but one female subject kept them caged. Seventy-five percent of the recipients bought substantial numbers of knickknacks for the birds. One of them built a remarkable playground for his budgie.

Although television ownership had no detectable effect on response to the questionnaire, ownership of budgies did. The subjects showed consistent improvement, as determined by their responses to the questionnaire, particularly on items that concerned attitudes toward people and toward the subject's own psychological health. The interviewers noted that people who owned budgies had formed a surprisingly intimate attachment to these birds given to them as a gift. The birds had become an important topic for conversation that displaced the monotonous concern for their own medical problems. The budgies were a social lubricant with friends, family, and neighbors who came to visit. One elderly woman found young children visiting far more often than before, and she amused visitors by teaching her budgie to recite their names. For the majority of the subjects, the budgies became a pleasurable personality in their private lives; it was not just a surrogate feathered human replacement.

Another example of the appeal and influence of a bird can be illustrated by Orman, a lame pigeon, who was the favorite "game" to be checked out of a summer recreation program in a park in Portland, Oregon. Orman enjoyed the company of people, especially in an advanced dancing class. In the class he created dance movements of his own while the dancers were developing theirs. The adaptability and learning ability of even a handicapped bird could suit it to the role of special companion in a home for the elderly (Kirkendall, 1973, and personal communication, 1973).

Even though we can't fully explain the beneficial effect of companion animals on human health and well-being, the mode of treatment is relatively inexpensive and has few risks, fewer than most of the therapeutic agents utilized today (Bustad et al., 1976b, c; Friedmann, 1979). We hope that sound and comprehensive studies in the near future will provide important answers to the questions now being raised about pet therapy.

Animals as Aids

Animals offer not only therapeutic assistance, but tangible help to people (see Wolff, 1970). Programs that train dogs to aid the handicapped have been operating for over 50 years and continue to expand. Guide dogs that assist the blind are a familiar sight to most of us. More recently, dogs have been specially trained to assist the hearing impaired and the physically handicapped. Summaries of existing programs are given in Appendix A.

The program to place dogs with the hearing impaired is relatively new. About 6% of our population have a hearing impairment, and about 14% of these (1.8 million people in the United States) are totally deaf. I was privileged to accompany Laura Rhea, counselor for the American Humane Association Training Program, in the follow-up of a placement of a hearing-trained dog. The recipient was a charming lady who lived alone, having raised a large family, and whose husband had recently died. Laura had placed the dog on a Saturday and had made contact with the local veterinarian regarding special needs and problems that might arise. I accompanied her on a follow-up on the third day after placement. As soon as we knocked on the door, we could hear the dog inside running to the door. Immediately the dog notified its owner of our presence, and led her to the front door. We were welcomed and had an interesting visit. The dog, whose name is Ranger, doesn't bark but places his paws on persons to communicate with them and get their attention. During this visit, Ranger's owner lay down on her bed, and Laura played a tape recording of a smoke alarm. On hearing it, Ranger leaped on the bed on top of its mistress. After she rose, the dog came into the living room and jumped on us.

Next, Laura tested the dog's response to a telephone ring. The dog did not respond but looked puzzled at the tape recorder, perceiving that the sound was not coming from the telephone and was of inferior quality. Dogs can detect very small changes in pitch. The acuity or preciseness of a dog's hearing was shown by the work of Pavlov when he trained dogs to come for their feed by striking middle C on a tuning fork. After they were well trained, he found C sharp or C flat or any other note varying by more than 8 vibrations from middle C produced no response in the dogs (Trew, 1949). Laura was told that Ranger was not responding to an alarm clock. Testing the alarm, we found that a buzzer and not a bell rang. Ranger had been trained for a bell. When Laura Rhea used her own alarm clock, the dog immediately responded.

Hearing dogs now have the same legal status as guide and seeing eye dogs in many states; we hope this will be true soon in all states. The hearing dogs are identifiable by a bright orange color and orange leash. Governor Dixy Lee Ray in Washington gave hearing dogs special legal status as soon as she learned about them. (Such recognition should also be extended to dogs that aid the handicapped.) Assistance dogs not only help their new owners, but can become essential and trustworthy companions.

Horses, too, are taking their place as special helpers for the handicapped. Therapeutic horseback riding was actively promoted in Britain after the 1947 poliomyelitis outbreak when many people were confined to hospitals for extended periods of time. Simultaneously, ingenious people in England and in

Norway decided that the routine and boring exercises required of the patients could be more appropriately done on a pony's back. This new approach became very successful, and an Advisory Council on Riding for the Disabled was formed in 1964 in Britain. This function was transferred in 1969 to the Riding for the Disabled Association. By 1971, 150 groups in Britain and five other countries were represented at the association's annual meeting (Highet, personal communication, 1979). The North American Riding for the Handicapped Association, Inc. was recently formed in the United States, and over 75 centers are operating (see also Williams, 1971).

People with many types of disabilities appear to be greatly aided by regular riding under the supervision of specially trained equestrians. In addition to emotional and social benefits from animal contact and learning to ride, significant improvement occurs in physical well-being, including balance, coordination, and mobility. This has certainly been the experience with epileptic patients at Bethel (Figure 16) in Bielefeld, Germany, as well as many other places (Bustad, 1978b; Funke and Hocke, personal communication, 1977; Simons, 1974). Instructors at the Little Bit Special Riders Program in Woodinville, Washington, are now in the process of quantifying improvements in their disabled students brought about by riding. Such quantitative evaluation will be a major goal of the Partnership in Equine Therapy and Education program now being established at Washington State University (WSU).

Not only the handicapped, but also many healthy older people could benefit by riding horses and affiliating with therapeutic riding clubs. I witnessed the joy of an 85-year-old aunt who resumed riding a horse after not riding for 40 years. The horse she is holding is the same equivalent age; both are alert and spirited, but gentle (Figure 17).

People no longer licensed to drive automobiles would gain great satisfaction from learning to ride a horse or to drive a horse-drawn cart. Horses provide a means of transportation in many locations, such as small towns or retirement homes, for older people, and allow them a greater degree

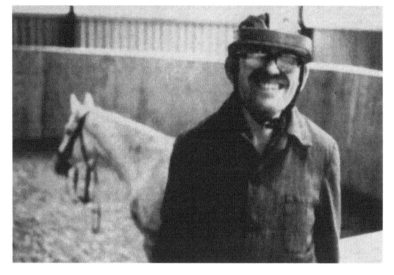

Figure 16. An elderly epileptic with a horse at Bethel (courtesy F. Höche).

Figure 17. Aunt Vinnie by her horse.

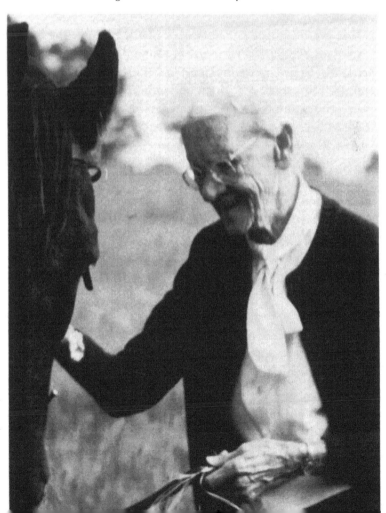

of independence in shopping, visiting, and attending church. At WSU, we are developing a program in riding and driving for the handicapped and elderly. Special seats are to be constructed in a modified jog cart that will provide a comfortable and safe means of getting into and out of the cart without climbing.

Community-Wide Animal Programs

Efficient and effective use of companion animals can be aided immensely by a concerted, cooperative community enterprise. Our experience in Pullman, Washington, and Moscow, Idaho (two towns only 8 miles apart) may help other communities in such an effort.

The WSU College of Veterinary Medicine took the lead in forming a People-Pet Partnership Council for our geographic area. The agencies represented on the Council include the county Epton Society (for the handicapped), area convalescent centers, university student counseling center and office for physically impaired students, departments of psychology and of physical education (therapeutic recreation), councils on aging, public schools, the College of Veterinary Medicine at WSU, the Student Chapter of the American Veterinary Association, and Cooperative Extension and the Department of Animal Sciences in the College of Agriculture WSU. We believe our program could serve as a model, with appropriate adaptation, for similar programs elsewhere.

This broadly based program has a number of long-range objectives:

- The education of school children and others about the responsibilities of pet ownership and the potential of pets for enriching their lives
- The utilization of animals in therapy for the physically, mentally, and emotionally handicapped
- The promotion of pets and companionship programs for the elderly, the lonely, students in dormitories, persons in nursing homes and prisons, and others

• The establishment of a referral system to enable area residents to obtain specially trained pets (for example, hearing dogs for the hearing impaired)
• The establishment of a clearinghouse to provide information on pet programs and to link resource people with persons wishing assistance in the area of utilization of pets
• The formation of a consultant group that will work with those who have specific people-pet problems.

Eventually, we hope that our specially trained advisers can serve as demonstrators and resource persons to state-wide agencies and institutions. Our objectives are being accomplished by cooperative interaction between skilled volunteers and agencies in our community. In monthly meetings, council members learn about the animal-people relationship and take specific action to accomplish the program's objectives (Bustad, 1978a, 1979a, c, d).

Community programs to promote pets as companions or therapeutic agents can take many forms. A Pet-a-Care Program was developed by the San Francisco Society for the Prevention of Cruelty to Animals. To be eligible for the Pet-a-Care program, the person must be 65 or over and have an annual income not exceeding $5,000. The Pet-a-Care program provides for every kind of veterinary service: visits, examinations, vaccinations, spaying and neutering surgery, hospitalization, even transportation to the hospital for the pet, for two dollars per treatment. The SPCA membership takes care of the rest of the expenses. It provides veterinary service for up to two pets per household. This makes it possible for old people with a low income to keep their pets. This same organization is moving to obtain changes in standard lease agreements so that senior citizens' building units will allow pets. Recently the Vincent Astor Foundation awarded a $250,000 grant to the Animal Medical Center in New York City to endow the Center's program of free care for pets of the elderly poor.

A group offering an assortment of healthy animals, including specially trained ones, can be a very useful service to any community. Such a proposed resource could be a modification of one described by Arkow of the American Humane Association called the Rent-a-Pet program (1973). This program emphasizes a loan procedure for small laboratory animals (gerbils, guinea pigs, hamsters, and rabbits) in schools. No charge is made for the service; in fact, cages and some supplies are furnished, and the animals are often retrieved during vacations, holidays, and weekends so adequate care is assured. Other forms of "pet banks" have been suggested (Walster, 1979; see also Arkow, 1976, 1977).

A Pet Animal Loan Service (PALS) could include some specially trained animals, as well as the usual pets. Demonstration animals could be taken to public and private institutions, and to individuals (for example, disabled and elderly). A specialist in animal training would introduce animals on a short-term basis in locations in which animals have potential for benefiting people's health and well-being. This specialist could also consult on selection of appropriate animals and the care and training of animals already in place. We believe this resource person should serve state institutions and qualify for support from state mental health offices. The program would emphasize the elderly, whether in their own homes or in group housing.

The idea of taking animals into institutional settings has become reality in several places. Frances Arnold, Director of Humane Education for the Berkeley-East Bay Humane Society, began over 10 years ago to visit nursing homes in her area. Well-trained animals, especially her dog Rags, perform an assortment of tricks and relate well to the rabbit, Brownie, and to the guinea pig, Spot. She would visit the day room of a nursing home, for example, and introduce the residents to her friends. She would give a short discourse on these animals, and then hand them around to the patients. The dog would visit each person on his own. The visit always brought a favorable reaction from the patients, many of whom wished to keep the animals (Jernigan, 1973; Levinson, 1970). This program could be initiated elsewhere to bring welcome variety into the lives of persons in institutions.

In 1976 the Massachusetts Society for the Prevention of Cruelty to Animals (MSPCA), along with the American Humane Education Society (AHES), with the cooperation of the Junior League of Boston, initiated a joint project to place well-behaved dogs and cats and other animals, such as rabbits, in eligible nursing homes for adoption. The MSPCA/AHES staff and community professionals train Junior League volunteers in pet therapy and problems of the elderly. The Junior League volunteers then introduce the pet therapy concept to the administrators and staff of the nursing homes. The animals are carefully selected from the animal shelter. They have to be one year or older and are screened for their temperament, maturity, training, and personality. The Angell Memorial Animal Hospital offers free neutering, a thorough medical examination, and the first year's routine medical care for these animals. After the animals are placed in a nursing home, Junior League volunteers continue to work with the animal, as well as the residents and administration, for at least a year. The program has been very successful. Some people who were uncommunicative have responded to the animals. The pets often rekindle warm memories of other pets and other times. The unabashed affection that these animals manifest and receive is socially acceptable and therapeutic (Kearny, 1977).

The Humane Society of Hennepin County in Minnesota initiated a program in the early seventies that involved sending letters to all physicians in the Twin City area inviting them to participate. Included in the letter was this statement, "If you have a patient you feel will be helped by the companionship of a pet or if you feel that the responsibility of having a pet will be helpful to your patient or that a pet will assist your patient's recovery in any way." They also included prescription blanks similar to those utilized by physicians. Figure 18 shows a copy of the "prescription."

The blanks were imprinted with the Society's name and

The Animal Humane Society
of HENNEPIN COUNTY
845 France Avenue North, Minneapolis 55422 • Telephone 522-4325

Pets by Prescription

NAME OF PATIENT _____ AGE _____

ADDRESS _____ PHONE _____
type of pet requested to be donated by Animal Humane Society:

R _____
(dog or cat, suggested sex, age or breed)

COMMENTS _____

DOCTOR'S SIGNATURE _____ PHONE _____

Figure 18. Hennepin County Humane Society
prescription form.

address. They had a space for the name of the person, comments by the physician, and his signature. The Society filled the prescription free of charge to the patient. Although the greatest attraction was for youngsters, the society encouraged older people to take advantage of the program. They felt that the family physician would know the most about a family's ability to take responsibility for the pet so that it would receive regular care and adequate food. Thus, neither pet nor patient would suffer from the relationship.

The variety of pet therapy and companion animal programs that can be introduced in communities is limited only by the resource people available and their ingenuity. However, since these programs are meant to have profound impact on people, certain principles should be observed in their introduction.

• Call a meeting of as many potential resource persons as

possible. With their help, assess the needs and potential in your community.

* Begin with a few programs that can be done thoroughly and that have provision for long-term continuation (both financial and manpower commitments).
* Continually assess progress toward stated objectives. Modify the program as needed. Establish a sound basis for evaluation.
* Let others know about your work so that they can benefit from your experiences.

Evaluative Instruments

Before the full potential of pets as companions and therapeutic agents can be realized, we must develop better evaluative tools for the situation, owner, and pet. A thorough study must be made of any situation into which a companion animal would be brought, whether a home or an institution. The following checklists could be completed by placement personnel. These checklists and other profiling instruments in this chapter are being developed by members of the People-Pet Partnership Council and should be regarded as preliminary drafts to be tested and modified. Research on these instruments will be undertaken through the Council, and data will be collected (Bustad, 1979b).

Interviewing Guide for Pet Placement
With Individuals

Instructions

If a pet is to be placed with an individual, then the following structured interview should be conducted by the person representing the agency responsible for selecting and placing a pet. The interviewer should arrange an appointment and spend the first few minutes of the interview establishing rapport with the individual. The interview should be held in the home of the interviewee with no others present. If a pet is to be used in a therapeutic situation, this interview should be augmented with comments from the consulting doctor/therapist concerning the reasons for recommending a pet and the type of pet suggested.

Pet and Personal History

1. Name: _____
   (last name)   (first name)   (middle initial)

2. Address: _____

   _____

3. Sex: _____

4. Year of birth: _____

5. Have you ever had a pet before? Yes _____ No _____.
   If yes, please describe the type of pet, and the age at which you had the pet, for any pet which you feel was important in your life.

   Type of Pet   Your Age

   _____   _____

   _____   _____

   _____   _____

   _____   _____

   _____   _____

   _____   _____

6. Please describe what you feel is the most important reason for keeping a pet, based upon your experience with pets:

   _____

   _____

Pet Placement

7. Do you live alone _____ or with others _____ (please check one response)?

8. If you live with other people, are these people in favor of

having a pet in the household? Yes _____ No _____
Comment:

9. Please describe your dwelling (for example, private home or apartment, etc.): _____
How long do you plan to live here? _____
10. Does the size of your dwelling (or the owners if rented) place any restrictions on the size of pet you would consider? Yes _____ No _____
If yes, please describe: _____
_____

11. What is the maximum amount of money you could spend to purchase a pet? _____
care for a pet, per month? _____
12. Are there any specific types of pets which would be unacceptable to you? Yes _____ No _____
If yes, please describe: _____
_____

13. Do you have any allergic conditions affected by particular animals? Yes _____ No _____
If yes, please describe: _____
_____

14. What proportion of your day is spent at home? _____%
15. Do you live in an urban _____, suburban _____, or rural _____ environment? (check one)
16. Do you have any disabilities or health conditions that might limit your ability to care for or manage a pet?
Yes _____ No _____
If yes, please describe: _____
_____
_____

17. Do you want access to a pet at all times or would a visiting pet be acceptable to you? _____
_____

18. Would you like more than one pet? Yes _____ No _____
    If yes, what combinations? _____

19. Do you wish to make a long-term _____ or short-term _____ commitment to a pet? (check one)

20. Would you prefer an active _____ or a quiet _____ pet? (check one)

21. Would you like follow-up visits by the person placing the pet? Yes _____ No _____
    If yes, monthly _____, weekly _____, or other _____

22. Do you have any worries or concerns about caring for a pet? Yes _____ No _____
    If yes, please describe: _____
    _____
    _____

23. What is the main reason you would like a pet?
    _____
    _____
    _____
    _____
    _____
    _____

Interviewing Guide for Pet Placement With an Institution

Instructions

The following structured interview should be conducted by the person representing the agency responsible for selecting and placing a pet in a nursing home, school, prison, or other institutional setting. The interviewer should arrange an appointment to speak individually with the professional workers—owner, teacher, director—as well as some of the residents, and spend the first few minutes of the interview establishing rapport. The interview should be held in a private

place with no others present. If a pet is to be used in a therapeutic situation, this interview should be augmented with
comments from the consulting doctor/therapist concerning
the reasons for recommending a pet and the type of pet
suggested.

Background

1. Name of Institution:_____

2. Address:_____

_____

3. Type of Institution:_____

4. Number and ages of residents:_____

_____

5. Number of staff members:_____

6. Has the institution ever housed pets before?
   Yes_____ No_____
   If yes, please describe the pets, list the dates the pets were
   kept, and comment on the residents' and staff members'
   feelings about the pets. (Use extra pages as required).

   Type of pet   Dates (years)   Comments

   _____

   _____

   _____

7. Description of your facility, especially the space available
   for the pet(s):_____

   _____

   _____

8. Areas where pet(s) would not be allowed:_____

   _____

9. Amount of money available to purchase pet(s):_____
   to maintain pet(s), per month:_____

10. Personnel for pet care; day:_____
    night (if applicable):_____
    vacations (if applicable):_____

11. Time available each day to care for pet(s):_____

12. Please describe what you think is the most important reason for keeping a pet in your institution:_____

_____

_____

_____

13. Have any residents or staff expressed positive feelings
about acquiring pet(s)? Yes_____ No_____
Number of residents_____ staff_____
Species suggested_____
Summary of comments_____

14. Have any residents expressed negative feelings about ac-
quiring pet(s)? Yes_____ No_____
Number of residents_____ staff_____
Species objected to_____
Summary of comments_____

15. Are there any specific types of pets which would be unacceptable to you? Yes_____ No_____
If yes, please describe_____

16. Do residents have any allergic conditions affected by particular animals? Yes_____ No_____
If yes, please describe_____

17. Do residents have disabilities which would affect the
choice of pet(s)? Yes_____ No_____
If yes, please describe_____

18. Do you want more than one pet? Yes_____ No_____
If yes, please describe combinations_____

19. Do you want access to a pet at all times, or would a visiting pet be acceptable?_____

20. Do you wish to make a long-term_____ or a short-
term_____commitment to a pet?
21. Would you prefer an active_____ or a quiet_____ pet?
22. Describe any worries or concerns you may have about
keeping a pet in the institution:_____

_____

_____

_____

23. Would you like follow-up visits by the persons placing a
pet? Yes_____ No_____
If yes, weekly_____, monthly_____, other_____
24. What arrangements can you make for the health care of a
pet?_____

_____

The profile of the pet should be matched with a profile of
the prospective owner (see Cattell and Korth, 1973). If one is
gentle and soft-spoken, it may not be appropriate to get a
large dog that requires some assertiveness. If one, however, is
very firm and aggressive, choosing a sensitive animal may not
be the appropriate selection. However, each choice must be
evaluated separately. A quiet person may benefit from having
a dog that develops assertiveness in the owner. Conversely, an
aggressive but aware owner may be gentled by having to train
a sensitive animal. Reputable breeders are a very good source
of information about what may be expected from a particular
breed or strain.

A self-evaluation of the potential owner's personality is
helpful. The following research instrument being developed
by Wong et al. (1977) could provide such a profile (Table 9).
This instrument is designed to be used before the animal is
selected, to assist in selection, and after the animal has been
with the owner for a period of time to evaluate its effect on
the owner's personality as the owner perceives it.

Table 9. Human Personality Profile (Modified from Wong, Greenfield, and Grubman, 1977 and from J. J. Sherwood, Ph.D. Dissert., 1962, *Self-Identity and Self-Actualization: A Theory in Research,* Univ. of Mich.: Ann Arbor.)

Self-Confident	└┴┴┴┴┴┴┘	Not Confident
Tolerant	└┴┴┴┴┴┴┘	Intolerant
Reserved	└┴┴┴┴┴┴┘	Outgoing
Participant	└┴┴┴┴┴┴┘	Nonparticipant
Authoritarian	└┴┴┴┴┴┴┘	Democratic
Competent	└┴┴┴┴┴┴┘	Incompetent
Nonaggressive	└┴┴┴┴┴┴┘	Aggressive
Honest	└┴┴┴┴┴┴┘	Dishonest
Passive	└┴┴┴┴┴┴┘	Active
Likable	└┴┴┴┴┴┴┘	Not Likable
Cooperative	└┴┴┴┴┴┴┘	Uncooperative
Self-Insight	└┴┴┴┴┴┴┘	Lack Insight
High Morality	└┴┴┴┴┴┴┘	Low Morality
Follower	└┴┴┴┴┴┴┘	Leader
Timid	└┴┴┴┴┴┴┘	Bold
Individualist	└┴┴┴┴┴┴┘	Conformist
Affectionate	└┴┴┴┴┴┴┘	Cold
Relaxed	└┴┴┴┴┴┴┘	Tense
Intelligent	└┴┴┴┴┴┴┘	Unintelligent
Conservative	└┴┴┴┴┴┴┘	Liberal
Friendly	└┴┴┴┴┴┴┘	Unfriendly
Independent	└┴┴┴┴┴┴┘	Dependent
Conventional	└┴┴┴┴┴┴┘	Unconventional

Instructions

1. Please indicate the location on the scale where you presently picture yourself by a P. Do not be concerned if you see yourself as being different in different situations, e.g., cooperative—independent: You are to indicate how you picture yourself in general or most usually.

2. Please indicate the location on the scale where you aspire to picture yourself in the next two years by an A. We are interested in the aspirations that people have for themselves. All persons have a desired picture of themselves

toward which they see themselves to be realistically striving. This is not meant to be your ideal—rather, that picture of yourself that you actually aspire to attain in the future. The scale runs continuously from one labeled extreme to the other, with the varying degrees being indicated by vertical lines.

Please mark both a P indicating your present picture of yourself and an A for your aspired picture in the appropriate space on the scale.

This profile should be completed by the prospective owner, or by a social worker or other trained person in situations where a pet may be used in therapy.

Persons selecting animals for therapy or companionship should consider the size, species, sex, age, temperament, and care required of a given type of animal. In the case of dogs and cats, an adult animal is recommended in most situations, especially if a well-trained one is available. However, if one has a great deal of time and is home continuously, it is rewarding to obtain and train a young animal. Simply choosing a breed for its appearance or to continue a breed tradition in the family is not necessarily the recommended approach. However, some people may need to obtain a handsome, purebred animal, so that they can display it with pride and talk about it with confidence.

In the case of the dog, one must realize that many behavior patterns are inherited and that specific breeds have been developed for efficiency and capability, often for certain tasks. It is a mistake to obtain a dog which has been specially bred for one purpose and then try to develop some other trait that may be difficult for the breed to master. It is possible to train almost any dog for almost any task, but not always efficiently. Through many centuries, over 400 breeds have been developed worldwide to accomplish certain tasks: hunting, guarding, herding, trailing, pulling large loads, or sitting on laps (Ensminger, 1977). This feature should be an aid in selecting animals (see also Brace, 1962).

Since behavior patterns and temperament may be inherited and selection can be made for specific behavior patterns, some animals logically could be bred for use with the handicapped and in animal-facilitated therapy. This endeavor needs careful investigation. Some recommendations have been made regarding choice of an animal for a particular situation, such as a hospital (Cooper, 1976).

Wild species should not be considered for use as companion animals. This restriction should also apply to the sale of wild species raised in captivity such as bobcats, large cats, coyotes, opossums, nonhuman primates, raccoons, or wolves. Wild species do not make suitable pets; they may be the source of zoonotic disease that can affect people, as well as our domestic population. Such animals cannot be fully trusted and removing them from their wild habitat in some cases disturbs the ecology of the area from which they originate.

In selecting animals for use as companions or for therapy situations, we must be very aware of the animal's well-being and minimize the chance of physical and mental trauma to the animal. The first step is to develop criteria for selecting the appropriate animal for a particular person and condition. A comprehensive profile of each animal being considered would enable evaluation of the animal's potential in various situations. A preplacement profile could also aid in assessing the impact of the experience on the animal.

The evaluative instruments presented here for profiling dogs and cats are useful for mature animals. (A guide for selection of a puppy or kitten is given in Appendix B).

Many people have worked with me and with Linda Hines, director of the People-Pet Partnership Council, to develop animal temperament profiles. They include Terry Ryan (dogs), Kaia Soren, Carol Baker, and Dr. Richard Ott (cats), and consultants to the PPP Council including Drs. Dudley Klopfer, Carroll Meek, Gus Kravas, and Marie Zeglen. This series of elimination tests is for animals over one year of age that are being considered as companion or therapeutic animals in institutions or individual homes. The tests are preliminary and must be refined in use by testing a variety of animals. Ideally the same animal should be tested on different days by a variety of people (male/female, old/young). The tester should carefully read and be familiar with the testing instrument. Also, it is assumed that the animal will have undergone a thorough physical examination to determine its health, including hearing ability, and arrangements will have been made to have it neutered.

It should be noted that neither tail movement nor ear position is used in evaluating dogs, since various breeds have different ways of normally holding the tail and ear. For example, "up" is not the normal tail position for every breed. German Shepherds almost never carry their tails "up." "Normal" for them is following the curve of their hind legs when standing; while gaiting, they hold the tail level with the back. Only a dominant German Shepherd who has been challenged or otherwise stimulated (when a male is "studdish," for example) will carry the tail "up" and then only briefly. It is also difficult to determine in some dock-tail breeds what they are trying to express with their tails. The tester should be aware that a wagging tail does not always indicate a friendly dog. Wagging can also be a sign of nervousness. Some "protection" trained dogs wag their tails furiously while attacking (Ryan, personal communication, 1979).

Position of the ears is also not easy to judge as a reliable body language trait. There are so many variables that it would be easy for a tester to misinterpret the dog's signal. On a prick-eared dog, laying the ears back is a sign of fear. An attacking dog also lays his ears back, perhaps to protect them. Many friendly prick-eared dogs will lay their ears back, even though they are not afraid or about to attack. Perhaps they are anticipating being petted and are getting them out of the way. Dogs with flop ears are very expressive with their ears, but it may be difficult to interpret the various positions (Ryan, personal communication, 1979).

CANINE SELECTION PROCEDURES

Test 1: Initial Observations

Allow the dog to investigate the testing area on its own. A room or fenced yard with minimal distractions is appropriate. The tester, in ordinary street clothes, enters the area and stands still, observing the dog for approximately 15 seconds. Record below the very first responses:

Acceptable:

_____Holds ground
_____Approaches tester
_____Hackles normal
_____Flews normal
_____Sniffs tester

_____

_____

Questionable:

_____Retreats
_____Crouches
_____Hackles up
_____Flews "puffing"
_____Moves about "stiff-legged"
_____Growls
_____Barks

_____

_____

Other observations:

_____Avoids eye contact
_____Stares at you
_____Whines
_____No response

_____

_____

Test 2: Approach to Dog

After initial, brief observations, approach the dog with hand extended, palm and fingers pointed downward. Do not "rush" in, but do not approach dog in a cautious or apprehensive manner. Walk up to the dog in a normal stride until your hand is within 6 to 12 inches of the dog's nose. Say nothing, and wait for the dog to make the next move.

Acceptable:

_____Extends head or steps forward to sniff hand

_____Seeks attention by nudging or leaning into hand

_____Acts playful by barks or actions

_____Licks hand

_____

_____

Questionable:

_____Turns head away or tries to ignore hand

_____Pulls back or retreats

_____Growls

_____Raises hackles

_____Barks (not to be confused with playful barking)

_____Flews "puffing"

_____Overly exuberant

_____Bares teeth (don't confuse with grin)

_____

_____

Other observations:

_____Stares at you

_____Ears up

_____Ears down

_____No response

_____

_____

Test 3: Handling of Dog

If the dog has not been eliminated by Tests 1 and 2, attempt to pet the dog, starting with the top of the head. Use the same attitude described in Test 2. Then brush the dog and determine its overall response or specially sensitive areas.

Acceptable:

_____Enjoys the attention
_____Tries to make friends
_____Becomes playful
_____Enjoys brushing

_____

_____

Questionable:

_____Pulls back or retreats
_____Growls
_____Flews "puffing"
_____Raises hackles
_____Quivers
_____Barks
_____Cowers
_____Rolls over on back
_____Submissive urination
_____Snaps, bites
_____Overly exuberant (jumps up; not calm by end of test)
_____Shows white of eye
_____Overly sensitive to grooming of certain areas

_____

_____

Other observations:

_____Aloof
_____Meets you, but with head lowered, averted eyes
_____Attempts to lick your face

_____

_____

Test 4: Interacting with Dog

If the dog has not been eliminated by Test 3, interact with it for about five minutes. This interaction could include the following:

- Play ball or tug of war
- Walk away, sit on floor, and call dog
- Pick dog up, and place on your lap
- Put hand around muzzle
- Have a mirror, plank, or portable tunnel in the room, and encourage the dog to investigate it.

Rate the dog by your subjective impressions in the following categories:

TRAITS .... OBSERVATION
...................................No   Yes
.... |1|2|3|4|5|6|7|
Aloof .... |__|__|__|__|__|__|__|
(Maintains distance, self-assured)
Apprehensive .... |__|__|__|__|__|__|__|
(Anxious, fearful, shows alarm)
Assertive .... |__|__|__|__|__|__|__|
(Expresses own needs, noses, or paws for attention)
Calm .... |__|__|__|__|__|__|__|
(Tranquil, composed, not agitated)
Dignified .... |__|__|__|__|__|__|__|
(Noble, poised, manifests appropriate behavior and manner)
Extroverted .... |__|__|__|__|__|__|__|
(Interested in others and surroundings)
Exuberant .... |__|__|__|__|__|__|__|
(Unrestrained high spirits)
Gentle .... |__|__|__|__|__|__|__|
(Tame, easily handled)
Noisy .... |__|__|__|__|__|__|__|
(Barks, whines)

Playful .... |_|_|_|_|_|_|_|_|
(Willing to initiate or participate in fun and attention)

Responsive .... |_|_|_|_|_|_|_|_|
(Reacts to involvement, interacts readily with people)

Sociable .... |_|_|_|_|_|_|_|_|
(Enjoys being with people)

Suspicious .... |_|_|_|_|_|_|_|_|
(Cautious, distrustful)

Trusting .... |_|_|_|_|_|_|_|_|
(Confident with people)

Willing to be handled .... |_|_|_|_|_|_|_|_|
(Readily accepts body contact)

Test 5: Stability

These tests will help reveal the stability of the dog's temperament. You will need a helper.

1. While casually interacting with the dog, have your helper make a very loud noise without warning; for example, hitting a metal pan with a spoon. Also, see how the dog reacts to fast arm movements.

Acceptable:

_____Notices, but continues previous activity
_____Notices and investigates
_____Startles, but recovers quickly

_____
_____

Questionable:

_____Flees
_____Cowers
_____Trembles
_____Moves as if to attack

_____
_____

Other (explain):

_____

_____

2. While playing with the dog, pinch its ears or the webbing between its toes.

Acceptable:

_____Tries to get away, but shows forgiveness
_____Yelps, but is not aggressive
_____Trusts you and allows further petting

_____
_____

Questionable:

_____Growls
_____Snaps
_____Acts fearful
_____Acts distrustful

_____
_____

3. While the dog is playing with you and distracted, have your helper conceal himself or herself in a closet or behind a door. Lead the dog close to the hiding place and have the helper suddenly jump out at the dog. Record the dog's reactions.

_____

_____

4. Have your helper hide around a corner, out of sight, with a noisy utility or shopping cart. Walk with the dog toward the intersection, as the helper rolls the cart in front of the dog as close as possible. Record the dog's reactions.

_____

_____

5. Note if the dog urinates or defecates in the room.

_____Yes

_____No

Test 6: Manners

We are not attempting to obedience train the dog here, but to work with it briefly on a lead to be sure it will be under reasonable control during a brief visit to the prospective owner's home or institution. We can also gain insight into the trainability of the dog.

Equipment • The dog should be on a lead, preferably one of leather or cotton webbing. It should have a properly fitting collar. A leather buckle collar is probably acceptable for a small or gentle dog, but a larger or more exuberant dog may benefit from a slip collar, preferably a nylon slip collar rather than a "choke chain." If a slip collar is used, do not leave it on the dog while it is unattended.

The Sit-Stay • The dog is placed in a standing position at your left side. Its leash should be gathered in your right hand so there is just a little slack. Command the dog to sit. If you know the dog's name, use it before the command. At the same time, pull up and back on the leash and press down on the dog's hips with your left hand. Praise it for complying. Hold it in the sitting position for a few seconds, continuing the praise, and using the word "stay" occasionally. Release it after no longer than 15 seconds and praise it again. Be consistent with your release words; for example, use "O.K." Repeat this procedure once or twice, with rest and attention in between.

Heeling • With the dog sitting at your left side, the leash gathered up in your right hand, command "heel." Stepping out with your left foot, walk briskly around, encouraging it to stay in the area of your left leg. If it fights the leash, slow up and keep encouraging it with pats on your leg and kind words. If it moves ahead or lags behind, get it back into position, with little tugs and releases of the leash. Repeat the command now and then. When the dog is in position, be sure to praise it. The leash should never be taut. If the dog pulls on the lead, use the tug/release method, along with praise and encouragement until it complies.

Spend no more than 30 seconds on the heeling drill at a time. Repeat the exercise once or twice, with no more than one minute's rest and attention in between. Before beginning each time, place the dog into a sitting position for a few seconds by the method described under "Sit-Stay."

Observations

- Did the dog fight the lead? Yes _____ No _____
- Did it *start* to assume the heel position after several 30-second sessions? Yes _____ No _____
- Was it happy to sit, without struggle, even though you had to hold it in position? Yes _____ No _____
- Does it seem willing to please and cooperate? Yes _____ No _____
- Is the dog mannerly enough at this point for a half-hour visit? Yes _____ No _____
- Other comments:

_____

_____

Test 7: A Visit to the Prospective Home

If the dog performed satisfactorily on tests 1-6, it is ready to visit the home of the prospective owner(s). During the visit, the dog should meet all persons with whom it will have contact, that is, family members such as children and grandchildren, administrators and staff members of institutions. If small children will be around the dog, the dog's handler might want to bring a child who will be under his control for safety reasons. While traveling, and during a visit of one-half hour to one hour, observations should be made on the following:

Actions while riding in a car
Meeting the person
Meeting other pets or family members
Climbing steps
Reaction to unusual gait or appearance of person
Reaction to wheel chair and crutches
Willingness to investigate house (let dog off the lead)
Response to the doorbell
Actions while being handled by prospective owner

A decision should not be made to have a trial live-in period at this time. All the people involved need time to evaluate the situation for at least one day. If the dog needs obedience training, a decision must be made on who will do the training. You could place the dog and allow the new owner to train the dog with help. Some people might benefit from attending a public obedience class with their dog.

Special Considerations for Institutions

The dog should be taken to meet different types of people and should be around all of the equipment.
Observations should be made in the following areas:

Does dog have trouble on slippery hall floors?
Who is the person responsible for the care of the dog?
Does the person fully understand the job?
Will there be a "rule" about tidbits to the dog from patients?
Where will the dog sleep?
Will it have a place to call its own?
Discuss the possibility of a crate for times when the dog cannot be supervised, especially during the trial period.
Will one person be sure the dog is exercised regularly?
What facilities are there for the dog to be taken outdoors?
If there is no fenced area, perhaps a portable chain-link run

could be set up for when the staff are short of time to take the dog out under supervision.

Are there areas that are "off-limits" to the dog?

How will the off-limits be enforced?

Test 8: The Trial Period

Ideally, during the initial visit the dog should have encountered most of the daily situations. It should be made clear that the dog is being placed on a "trial" basis. People should not be made to feel guilty if the dog must be returned. They should be given the names of two contact persons and be encouraged to seek advice or help for any problem, however slight. The prospective owner should understand that the purpose of the one-month trial period is to see how the dog fits in.

As part of the introduction process, the prospective owner should be instructed in feeding, grooming, exercising, and caring for the dog. Check-ups by placement counselors in person should be made each week during the trial period.

FELINE SELECTION PROCEDURES

The cat should be taken from its cage by someone other than the tester and placed in a small room. The tester should wear ordinary street clothes (no white laboratory coat) and enter the room in a calm manner.

Test 1: Initial Observations

Observe the cat for one minute and write your observations.

_____Hides

_____Sits and looks at you

_____Explores the room—slinks

_____Explores the room—normal stance

_____Approaches or comes to you

_____Other, please specify_____

_____

Test 2: Interactions with Cat

Approach to about 5 feet, squat down, and call the cat.

_____Hisses

_____Does not come

_____Makes eye contact

_____Approaches slowly

_____Comes immediately

_____Other, please specify_____

_____

If cat does not come, call again and motion with your hands.

_____Hisses

_____Does not come

_____Makes eye contact

_____Approaches slowly

_____Comes immediately

_____

_____

Roll a ball across the floor.

_____No response

_____Watches ball

_____Follows ball

_____Attacks ball

_____

_____

Pick up the cat and sit in a chair. Put the cat on your lap, but do not pet.

_____Jumps off or other negative response

_____Sits there nervously

_____Sits there calmly

_____Seeks affection (meows, rubs, makes eye contact)

_____

_____

Stroke across the back from head to tail and then stop.

_____Jumps off or other negative response

_____Sits there nervously
_____Sits there calmly
_____Seeks affection (meows, rubs, makes eye contact)
_____Purrs

_____

_____

Scratch head, chin, and ears.

_____Jumps off
_____Tolerates scratching
_____Purrs

_____

_____

Cradle cat in your arms, on its back.

_____Tries to escape
_____Does not struggle
_____Purrs

_____

_____

Scratch its stomach while cradling in arms.

_____Tries to escape
_____Does not struggle
_____Plays
_____Purrs

_____

_____

Pinch a toe (ignore the involuntary response to withdraw the foot).

_____Hisses
_____Tries to escape
_____Does not struggle
_____Purrs

_____

_____

Hold cat on your lap. Using a grooming brush, stroke from head to tail.

_____Bites or scratches, tries to escape
_____Does not struggle
_____Purrs

_____

_____

Brush fur from tail to head.

_____Tries to escape, bite, or scratch
_____Does not struggle
_____Purrs

_____

_____

Put cat down on the floor. Wait until the cat is not watching you, then emit sudden noise.

_____Hides
_____Does not respond
_____Looks at you, seems disturbed
_____Looks at you, seems unaffected

_____

_____

Test 3: Temperament Profile for Cats

If the cat behaves in an acceptable manner for Tests 1 and 2, proceed to the temperament profile. Sit and play with or interact with the cat for 15 minutes to half an hour and then rate it.

TRAITS	OBSERVATIONS						
	No						Yes
	1	2	3	4	5	6	7
Affectionate							
(Seeks and/or enjoys attention)							
Aggressive							
(Approaches boldly, makes preferences known)							
Alert							
(Notices sounds, movements)							

Aloof. . . . . |__|__|__|__|__|__|__|
(Maintains distance, self-assured)

Apprehensive. . . . . |__|__|__|__|__|__|__|
(Anxious, fearful, feels alarm)

Calm . . . . |__|__|__|__|__|__|__|
(Tranquil, composed, not agitated)

Extroverted. . . . . |__|__|__|__|__|__|__|
(Interested in others and surroundings)

Gentle . . . . |__|__|__|__|__|__|__|
(Tame, easily handled)

Inquisitive . . . . |__|__|__|__|__|__|__|
(Investigates people, objects, sounds)

Playful. . . . . |__|__|__|__|__|__|__|
(Willing to initiate or participate in fun and attention)

Responsive . . . . |__|__|__|__|__|__|__|
(Reacts to involvement, interacts readily with people)

Vocal. . . . . |__|__|__|__|__|__|__|
(Meows, growls)

If the cat has performed acceptably on tests 1-3, it should be taken on a preliminary visit to the prospective owner's home and placed on a trial basis. See tests 7 and 8 in the canine selection test series.

Since these tests are in a preliminary stage, positive and negative scores cannot be assigned until more research has been done. Such research is now underway at Washington State University. Periodic rating of the animals is encouraged because changes occur as a result of attention, handling, and care. With more experience, more quantitative assessments may be possible. At this stage, only qualitative judgment on the basis of these tests can be used. Once extensive data have been gathered on a variety of animals, recommendations can be made regarding the temperament criteria that most accurately describe animals that can be placed successfully in specific situations. Evaluations are essential in measuring the success of the animal in a given situation. A carefully prepared preplacement evaluation should be made of the situation into which the animal will be placed. Postplacement evaluations to determine success in meeting specific goals should be conducted at regular intervals. Such evaluations should be of great value in advising other individuals or institutions on the selection of appropriate pets (see Hart, 1978).

Potential Problems

This discussion is not complete without addressing some of the problems one might encounter in the placement of animals and methods of dealing with them (see Brodie, 1979).

1. Disease: An assortment of diseases are transmissible from animals to people. The elderly and those in poor physical health may be especially susceptible to animal-transmitted diseases and infections. Any animal selected for older people must have a physical examination and must be healthy. Appropriate immunizations should be given animals before their introduction into any home for the aged.

2. Allergies: Some people have allergies or respiratory diseases that would preclude having an animal, at least in close proximity. A patient's history in this regard should be examined. Also, some patients have allergies only to certain animals or certain breeds of animals. Such allergies must be determined before any animal is introduced. In some institutions it may be appropriate to restrict animals to certain areas and quarters.

3. Physical injury: Dogs and cats bite and scratch, especially if the animals are not selected carefully and the owners are not instructed in how to handle them. Falls from horses or kicks by horses are also of concern. To minimize such problems, animals must be properly trained before their use by the elderly. Special training may be required, for example, for animals given to people who have difficulty walking and may trip over an animal. They should receive animals trained to avoid people so afflicted.

4. Public health aspects and sanitation: The presence of animals leads to problems of sanitation, particularly from biological waste, food, hair, dandruff, and secretions. Odors, too, can be a problem. Many institutions are, of course, prepared to

handle the problem of human elimination, and some of the same problems may occur with animals. However, animals can be trained to be very neat and clean. Special care must be taken to exclude animals from food preparation and dining areas, as well as in the intensive care units of institutions.

Noise pollution must also be considered. Dogs that incessantly bark or cats that make a great deal of noise, especially at night, should be retrained, replaced, or not introduced into an institution in the first place. Adequate facilities, too, must be developed for housing the animals. Sanitary, readily cleaned quarters for the animals, with plenty of room, are vital for any animals. Runs should be provided with flushing facilities and hot water for cleaning. The animals will keep themselves clean if their quarters are adequately maintained. Some animals require a great deal of attention relative to grooming. This need can have positive effects in that the patients in certain institutions may find that responsibility for bathing, brushing, and combing has therapeutic value. These considerations must be dealt with since grooming does contribute to having a clean animal that doesn't leave hair all over the quarters.

5. Reproduction and associated behavior: In most institutional settings and also in placement of animals with individuals, one must recognize that neutered animals tend to be more dependent, dependable, affectionate, gentle, and in general make better companions. Since they also tend to roam less and are more stable, greater longevity is likely. In a few selected locations, a cat might be allowed to have kittens as a part of therapy, but these instances would be limited.

6. Animal abuse: Some patients in institutions and certain individuals may take out their aggressions and frustrations on an animal. In this regard, the prospective owners must be evaluated regarding the possibilities of their abuse of animals, and the proper animal should be selected for them. In some cases, close supervision may be necessary. Education of the individuals before the introduction of animals is important in preventing such abuse.

7. Rejection: Rejection could be a problem in animal-facilitated therapy. If the animal rejects or appears to reject the person that it is supposed to aid, one must determine whether this is only an initial reaction or whether a mismatch exists between the patient and animal companion. A different problem arises if, after the acceptance of an animal by a given person, this person concentrates only on the animal and rejects people, thus losing opportunities for social exchange. In Corson's work at the Castle Nursing Home, in Phil Arkow's observations in a review of the literature, in Mugford's observations (1979b), and in our own experience, this has not been a serious problem. Usually the animal increases social exchange and has a positive effect on other residents and patients in an institutional meeting. It opens pathways to friendship.

A related difficulty is that a person who is to leave an institution where close association has developed with an animal may experience a deep depression or a "parting problem." Usually the pet has a strengthening effect on a person's self-reliance and psychological well-being, according to Corson. Therefore, it is certainly worthwhile to consider arranging for the patient to be provided with a suitable pet before departing to a new situation (Quinn, personal communication, 1979).

8. Financial responsibilities: Animals brought into homes or institutions do cost money, although volunteer assistance is readily available for acquiring animals and for instructing people in handling and caring for them. Veterinarians often contribute their services for at least some of the health care. The patients should be given an opportunity to contribute to providing for the animals, not only in the care but also in the financial arrangements. Many of them are pleased to be able to contribute to various aspects of the companion animal program.

9. Legal liability: The various liabilities that can result from accidents and injuries must be discussed and appropriate insurance obtained. This is especially true with larger animals and disease problems. The local and state health department

ordinances and regulations, the sanitation codes, and animal bans must be respected in each locale.

Although potential problems should be given consideration, a perspective must be maintained. Brickel (1979) reports very successful results in using cats in a hospital-based geriatric population. The cats stimulated positive interactions between patients themselves and between patients and staff. The animals suffered no physical damage and were very sensitive to disabilities of the patients. In general, the cats made the hospital setting more homelike and enjoyable. Daily time spent by staff per shift in caring for the animals averaged 8.6 minutes. Average cost for the care was 2.43 cents every day. The conclusion was that using pet mascots was valuable, economic and of minimal time cost to staff in the effort to improve the functioning of the patient population.

In a broader sense, some potential problems in using animals in a variety of situations are directly related to the question of responsibility of the animal owner (Beck, 1975). It is important that both individual and group owners of animals realize that owning an animal is not only an economic investment but a responsibility of great consequence. A first-time owner of an animal should attend classes and read information on animals and their care, handling, and proper training. In this regard, a qualification examination and permit to own animals may be a plan worthy of discussion and possible implementation. As companion animal owners, our responsibilities include thoughtfulness regarding our neighbors and their property. This extends to cleaning up our animal's droppings, obeying all leash laws, and doing our part in controlling overpopulation of animals. Assumption of all of these responsibilities would go a long way towards abatement of the many complaints about companion animals (see Joshua, 1974; Beck, 1975).

VETERINARY CARE

In routine care of supportive animals, it is important that fees are discussed candidly at the outset. Many veterinarians make special arrangements with elderly patients and nonprofit institutions for care of their animals. These veterinarians regard such assistance as a civic duty and responsibility (see Brodie, 1979). The veterinarian should also provide consultation on animal behavior problems, euthanasia, and grief following the death of an animal (Bustad, 1979a, c; Bustad and Hines, 1980; Goering, 1978; Keddie, 1979; Voith, 1979; Wallin, 1978).

Pet-A-Care Plan: There are some moves towards recommending a plan that would subsidize the cost of maintaining an animal. This health insurance could help especially those people who are old and cannot fully afford, but desperately need, an animal. Some modest assistance for providing for a companion animal that is vital to health and well-being would seem as justified as some of the costs now paid by Medicare. Such aid could include costs of obtaining and supporting seeing eye or hearing dogs, animals placed for health and security reasons, and pets vital as companions.

Pet Health Plans: For many years attempts have been made to promote voluntary hospitalization and animal health plans. The American Veterinary Medical Association has stated that such plans probably will become a reality in the form of prepaid veterinary hospital and clinic policies. It could be of great assistance to retired people owning pets and living on modest, fixed incomes. If such a plan is implemented, it is recommended that the pet owner be allowed the freedom to select the veterinarian.

CHAPTER 5

AFTERWORD

Animals have been of great assistance to us in understanding aging in people and in helping to clarify the complexities of some of our most costly diseases of the elderly. Animal studies have shown us how to alleviate some diseases by improved nutrition, modified life style, and animal companionship. Rather than emphasize the totally negative definitions of aging, I prefer to consider aging as the processes associated with attaining maturity. My friend Maggie Kuhn provides some perspective on these processes when she said: "Aging occurs from conception to resurrection." Old age can be a time of fulfillment, a period worthwhile in itself with its own share of joy and sadness. However, as the director of the National Institute of Aging, Dr. Butler, has expressed, in old age there is unique developmental work to be done. It is our responsibility as the elderly to clarify, deepen, and find use for what we have already obtained in a lifetime of learning and adapting.

While waiting for definitive studies to answer all of the questions posed in the introduction, the elderly can take definite steps to avoid or ameliorate the changes and diseases described in Chapters 2 and 3. Specifically, they can pay close attention to their diet and exercise.

Nutrition

For most of recorded history, many people have expressed the thought that we are what we eat. Diseases were thought to have been caused often by what was eaten and also were thought to be cured by dietary means. The Greek historian Herodotus in the fifth century B. C. stated that the Egyptians believed all diseases had their origin in food. In early Greece, Hippocrates (who is often regarded as the father of medicine) often prescribed particular diets as part of the treatment for his patients. He believed that good health was dependent on a particular combination of nutrients.

We have made some advances since the times of Herodotus and Hippocrates, but we haven't yet reached the point in our data bank that we can make firm dietary recommendations in all chronic conditions. In fact, after over two years of reviewing the literature for material in this book, it was distressing for me to realize that the only clear association between diet and chronic disease was that between alcohol and liver disease, salt and hypertension, and sucrose and dental caries (IN News, 1979). But there is some strong suggestive evidence that certain dietary components and elements of our life style are related to the induction, nature, incidence, and course of coronary heart disease, cancer, osteoporosis, and certain mental disorders. As a result of this evidence, a number of tentative recommendations are made and the bases for them are given. Some of them are admittedly like chicken soup—it won't do any harm and it might help.

The basis for most suggestions on individual intake of food are the recommended dietary allowances (RDA) of the National Academy of Sciences Food and Nutrition Board, which periodically updates their information. Although useful, RDA addresses the needs of a standard person age 25; these criteria hardly address the needs of an older person who may have one or more chronic diseases, who is no longer busily engaged in work, who may be very sedentary and who is often overweight (see Hegsted, 1975a, b; Harper, 1978). I have stressed that no average elderly persons exist. All people are unique, and diversity and uniqueness increase with age. This observation dictates an individual approach to each person as regards nutritional requirements and recommendations. Also, since physiological changes occur with time, the nutritional requirement should be reassessed periodically (see Bazzarre, 1978; Busse, 1978; Watkin, 1973).

Although the nutritional requirements of the elderly probably differ little from those who are younger, as a group the elderly seem to suffer much more from inadequate nutrition. Malnutrition among the elderly may be due to several factors. One of the most important is loneliness. In most instances, appetite decreases with lack of companionship (see Clarke and Wakefield, 1975; Creel, 1976). Our earliest recollections of food consumption involved body contact and subsequently our social life was built around food. Food consumption, it seems, is as much a social and psychological event as a biological one.

Elderly people, especially those who are for the first time living alone, may become apathetic and lose interest in preparing meals. Without adequate nutrition, they lack energy, are always tired, and become even more apathetic. The B vitamins along with vitamin C are depleted first because they are required daily. With vitamin depletion, mental confusion can occur and a worsened situation nutritionally and socially results. I recognized this vicious circle in my own life while a prisoner of war when I had inadequate nutrition. It required a great deal of motivation and self-discipline on my part to overcome the apathy of a malnourished state. We had to encourage one another to forage for food, even though it would have been easier to lie down and sleep. Had I been alone, as are many elderly, it would have been doubly difficult to overcome apathy and to expend waning energy to seek food.

When I turned 60 I wrote the following nutritional

prescription for my wife, my friends, and me in order to prevent malnutrition during the next couple of decades (see Todhunter and Darby, 1978; Truswell, 1978; Watkin, 1973; Weg, 1978; Weir et al., 1978). I also include some data that lend credence to my recommendations.

PROTEINS

The protein requirements of the elderly are generally similar to those of young adults if one uses lean body mass (muscle mass) rather than body weight (Zanni et al., 1979; see also Munro and Young, 1978). Since we eat less as we age, it is important that we obtain protein of very high quality. It is recommended that up to 20% of our caloric intake be protein. The protein should include milk or dairy products such as cheese. Cheese is a good substitute for those who have difficulty consuming milk because of flatulence or other reasons. Eggs are also an excellent source of protein. Many people have unfortunately given up eggs because of their cholesterol content. For a large segment of our population, there is little justification for not eating 3 to 5 eggs per week since this number of eggs do not appear by themselves to result in elevation of blood cholesterol and are a good source of protein (Porter et al., 1977; Kummerow et al., 1977; and see Truswell, 1978). Eggs should be evaluated in light of other dietary constituents.

Meat should be of high quality and include a variety of red and white meat. A reasonable protein allowance for those over 65 is about 2 grams per kilogram of their appropriate weight (Rao, 1973) but the amount and quality should be adjusted to the needs of the individual patient.

FAT

Fat for the elderly should be limited to 25 to 30% of the diet. This recommendation is made because in large amounts fat may reduce the consumption of carbohydrate and protein (which are sources of many of the necessary food components), and it may interfere with calcium absorption. The diet should contain the necessary fatty acids, especially linoleic.

Many people recommend that most of the fat be polyunsaturates. For special reasons, a physician may wish to include some polyunsaturates, but at the present state of knowledge, I hesitate to recommend hydrogenated oils with a high content of transfatty acid. Also, I believe butter (but not very much) is better than margarines that may contain more than 40, 50, or even 60% transfatty acid. A concerted effort should be made to require that the label on all products indicate the content of transfatty acids and to perform studies on their safety.

CARBOHYDRATE

About 55% of the diet should contain a wide variety of complex carbohydrate foods. This is recommended to provide the necessary vitamins, minerals, and fiber.

VITAMINS

Vitamin deficiency is likely in the elderly unless great care is taken to include all of the food groups mentioned here (Brin and Bauernfiend, 1978). If vegetables aren't added, then vitamin A may be missing. If fruits are not included, vitamin C will be low. If whole grain breads and cereals are not included, then B vitamins may be in short supply. Heat processed and convenience foods may be low in vitamin E (Lyons and Trulson, 1956: Pelcovits, 1972; Koehler et al., 1977). Vitamin D may be lacking if the individual is not exposed to sunlight.

Many medicinals can lead to vitamin deficiencies; in an early study by Jordan et al. (1954), it was shown that over half of the people took laxatives, which, of course, lead to rapid transit time of the intestinal content so that absorption is decreased. Mineral oil is a laxative that reduces the absorption of fat-soluble vitamins. Some antibiotics may reduce vitamin K availability, and anticonvulsant drugs may produce folic acid deficiency (Baisley et al., 1971). In view of these possible complications and shortages of vitamins, some supplementation, at least of vitamins B and C, is recommended. This should not, however, be excessive; money could be better spent to buy higher quality food (Mayer, 1974).

MINERALS

If the elderly person does not drink milk and has a low iron intake, low hemoglobin and serious loss of calcium from bone can result (Albanese, 1978). It is very important that high calcium intake be maintained throughout life. Dolomite is recommended by some for the elderly. I take it because I can't drink much milk. Salt intake should be reduced since it may contribute to congestive heart failure, hypertensions, cirrhosis of the liver, and retention of fluid (Mayer, 1974). Zinc deficiency can result if meat and cereals are not taken in sufficient supply; a zinc deficiency can lead to some impairment of taste and can also affect wound healing (Baisley et al., 1971). It is important that critical minerals be included in the diet daily.

FIBER

Whole grain cereals, vegetables, and fruits are recommended, if a person is able to eat these, since they have a laxative effect (Bass, 1977). Some fiber, but apparently not wheat bran fiber, is helpful in binding cholesterol, if that is considered to be a problem. The consensus of gastroenterologists at a 1977 conference was that high fiber foods, i.e., those that contain substantial cellulose, hemicellulose, pectin, and gums, may protect the colon from diverticulosis and cancer. Data conflict as to whether the toxicity of certain substances is reduced by binding properties of a high fiber diet, the change in the microbiological and chemical environment, and the change in intestinal transit time that may result. Certain high fiber foods may aggravate constipation due to spastic colon and cause deficiency in some trace elements (Sandstead et al., 1979; Cummings, 1978), but the effect on trace element loss is variable (Sandstead et al., 1978).

One possible advantage suggested for foods containing high amounts of dietary fiber (e.g., fruits, vegetables, and cereals) is that more bulk is thereby ingested so satiation occurs sooner than with items high in sugar. Caloric intake can thereby be reduced, and absorptive efficiency may be reduced with

high dietary fiber. Furthermore, food items high in dietary
fiber increase the amount of chewing, hence saliva and probably gastric juice, and increase the water intake, which may
be beneficial.

Chemical Constituents in the Diet

Many people, including many elderly, succumb to publicity
pleas to purchase 100% natural foods and get away from all
the artificial additives. But all living things are made up of
chemicals. Many people go to health food stores where the
food is often expensive because the food is alleged to have
more nutrients, thereby requiring less intake to remain healthy,
and thus really offering a bargain. The truth is that many substances in nature are far more toxic than any we've synthesized (see Report of Committee on Food Protection, NRC,
1973; Hall, 1977; Miller, 1973). Some are carcinogenic; others
may cause high blood pressure or a high incidence of goiter.
Eating or drinking a chemical is not hazardous unless it's
toxic—a poison. Additives, at least the ones with which I'm
familiar, have been submitted to extensive testing, while
many of the natural substances never have. In the final analysis, there really are no safe substances, just safe amounts. It is
generally accepted in scientific circles that the beneficial or
toxic effects of a given substance, whether derived from natural sources or synthesized in the laboratory, are identical.

Unfortunately, many people do not believe this, including
many of the elderly. As a result, the health food industry is
booming today. People's worries about side effects of food
additives, their preoccupation with body weight and worship
of all that is "natural" have combined to create a 1.5 billion-
dollar-a-year demand for an assortment of raw grains, "natural" vitamins, herbs, roots, an assortment of fibrous materials,
seed sprouts, and natural honey and sugar. The Federal Trade
Commission is considering a staff recommendation that the
word "health" be banned when associated with food. More
people are coming to realize that a product labeled "all natural" is not necessarily good for you.

I would hope that the elderly won't be taken in by the "raw kick," for example, raw fruits and vegetables, natural vitamins, raw sugar and honey, and raw milk. Cooking converts many fruits and vegetables to more digestible and nutritious products (as carrots, cauliflower, spinach). Many people can't eat raw apples but do well on applesauce. Raw sugar and honey are basically sugar—sources of calories. The extra nutrients present in honey and raw sugar are present in such minute amounts a person would have to eat horrendous quantities to benefit from their nutritional contribution. Refined sugar has been blamed for diabetes, cancer, and heart disease; the chief concerns with it appear to be that it offers empty calories, is somewhat addictive, is implicated in causing dental caries, and may tend to replace more important food items, e.g. fruits and vegetables. Pasteurization does not destroy the important nutrients of milk; it does, however, protect the consumer against disease-producing bacteria such as brucellosis (undulant fever), diphtheria, typhoid fever, and several others.

Finally, most natural vitamins are often really small portions of natural products blended with large amounts of synthetics. Each vitamin is a specific chemical compound, whether derived from food or synthesized. Our bodies probably use either one equally well. Excessive amounts of several vitamins are harmful. It is well to remember that many vitamins, along with many vital drugs originally derived from plants, are now chemically synthesized in order to provide an adequate supply for the health requirements of the world.

WATER

I recommend that elderly drink at least six glasses of water each day (Rao, 1973). Fruit juices can be substituted, of course.

CALORIC INTAKE

At least 1,500 calories is a recommended goal for many women and up to 2,400 for many men. The body weight of each individual is, of course, a good indication of proper intake, and daily weighing is a good habit. These caloric intakes would not be sufficient if the person is very active. Exercise, which is discussed next, is an important consideration. "Man soll die speisen nach der Bewegung und Starke des Leibes ab messen." (One should measure one's food according to one's activity and physique.) F. Hoffman (1715)

EXERCISE

Although anecdotal data are extensive on the value of exercise, definitive longitudinal studies in people to prove that the life span is extended by a certain exercise regimen throughout life have escaped my search. There are, however, sufficient data on people and animals to convince me that most people and animals would benefit from a life-long moderate exercise regimen. The best exercise may be work. Many people's physical activity may be limited during much of their careers. When I became 50, I began running, then walking and riding a bicycle so that 5 to 7 days a week my heart rate reaches at least 120. Vigorous walking is recommended for all elderly persons who are physically capable of walking. For some, a regimen of exercise in bed or in the water, as recommended by physical therapists, is helpful (Adrian, personal communication, 1979).

Dr. DeVries (1968) engaged a group of 70-year-old men in a one-year exercise program that seemed to improve their health and well-being. Almost everyone agrees that moderate exercise in the elderly slows calcium loss from bones, increases muscle mass, helps reduce body fat, increases aerobic power of muscles, and probably improves neurological functions. Violent exercise and occasional weekend-warrior activities are probably contraindicated for those with neuromuscular and cardiovascular malfunctions. It is important to keep the feet fit. Standing too long, running on pavement, and wearing ill-fitting shoes are to be avoided. In some cities, Preventicare groups are being formed to encourage exercise in the elderly, with some remarkable results (Robinson, 1980). More information on such programs is available from the Lawrence Frankel Foundation (Virginia at Brooks St., Charleston, S. Va. 25301).

Animal Contributions to the Aging

Animals contribute greatly to the physical and psychological well-being of people. This conclusion naturally follows from two important premises: People need to love and be loved, and they must feel needed. Animals provide companionship, love, and a reason for living for the aging and many other people, especially those left alone by the death of a mate. Animals give purpose to those undergoing rehabilitation, give aid to those with physical handicaps, and offer help to those who have physical ailments. Governmental assistance that would enable the elderly to keep animals at home would be a wise program, since animals provide clear benefits. The elderly will remain independent in their homes longer, and the cost is relatively small compared with that required for other types of companionship.

Animal-facilitated therapy is not a panacea for all the woes that plague mankind; but countless people's lives have been enriched by an assortment of feathered, finned, funny, or furred creatures.

Conclusion

The bright side of the picture depicting aging is that about 75% of those over 65 live in private residences and use the health care system that is utilized by everybody else. Although they may have an acute illness, they have many good years ahead of them, especially if we in geriatric medicine do our work. Physicians taking care of the people, and veterinarians and animal-care personnel ministering to their animals, will permit the elderly to remain independent in their homes longer and will thereby contribute to their happiness and health. Whatever happens, however, the delivery of medical care for the elderly must employ a multidisciplined approach (Yoxall and Yoxall, 1979; Bustad, 1979a).

One of the greatest contributions the elderly can make as grandparents and as teachers of our young is to convince them that modifying their lifestyle and their dietary habits early in life will result in a better and healthier later life. Rockstein and

Sussman (1976) estimated that approximately one-half to one-third of the health problems experienced by older individuals are believed to be directly or indirectly related to nutrition, most significantly in their early years. I believe, as they, that better nutrition early in life would have a remarkable effect on longevity and the quality of later life. A change in diet and mode of life will have practical consequences for millions of people who are coronary prone (Stamler, 1975). If the upcoming generations were introduced to new and better habits, we could see a dramatic reduction in overeating, sedentary living, cigarette smoking, and resultant decreases in commonplace hyperlipidemia, obesity, hypertension, hyperglycemia, hyperuricemia, and impaired cardiopulmonary function and probably hearing. By education and social change, with the cooperation and leadership of the older people, we can help change childhood and adolescent patterns of behavior including diet, exercise, coping with stress, and patterns of work and lifestyle. Combined efforts in behavioral and biomedical research will help us in this important endeavor.

I urge increased research support, from public and private sectors, with emphasis on basic research. During my lifetime, I have witnessed the control of most of the infectious diseases that have plagued people and animals for centuries (Spink, 1979). Some of the most basic research, though the goals were other than preventing polio or reducing the incidence of suffering and early demise of cardiac patients, helped us control polio and, in this decade, reduce deaths from heart attacks by about 40%. Thereby, the taxpayers saved billions of dollars. We now need millions of dollars in research to produce results that can save much of the billions of dollars now being spent on caring for those with heart disease, cancer, osteoporosis, periodontal disease, and mental disorders.

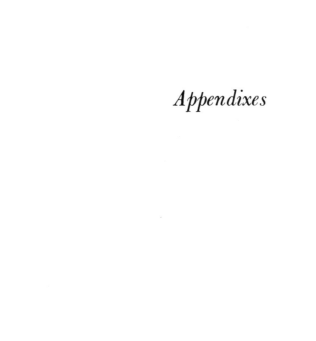

Appendixes

AGENCIES TRAINING DOGS TO AID THE HANDICAPPED

Visually Handicapped

GUIDE DOGS FOR THE BLIND

This program originated in 1942 when five women with the American Women's Volunteer Service in San Francisco organized the guide dog program for American servicemen who were blinded in World War II. In founding the program, they developed a training program for guide dogs, along with an in-residence training program for the blind person. Both the dog and training were provided free of charge to blind veterans. The program was later expanded to any qualified and deserving blind person and was relocated from Los Gatos to San Rafael, California.

The program uses three breeds of dogs: the golden retriever; the Labrador retriever, both black and yellow; and the German shepherd. These breeds, they feel, have proved to be most satisfactory in that they can adapt to hot and cold climates, are easy to groom, are of moderate size, and are willing workers. Their school has its own breeding stock, all within a 50-mile radius. However, they have been known to take a donated dog of exceptional pedigree. The pups are born at the school's kennels and stay with their mothers until they are six weeks old. The rejection rate has been reduced by a careful selection of breeding colony and breeding pairs (Pfaffenberger et al., 1976). From the age of six to eleven weeks, the pups go through a testing program, administered by volunteers, to determine their reaction to footings, obstacles, and any strange sounds, as well as their willingness and ability to learn.

At the end of the testing period, those animals that pass their initial tests are given to 4-H members in the western states. The dogs live with these members for 12 to 15 months because a socialization period in a family atmosphere is vital for the soundness of the dog. The 4-H youngsters teach the canines simple obedience, take them on family outings, give them plenty of affection, and also introduce them to many situations. In fact, in our town of Pullman they use our new Veterinary Science Building to accustom the animals to elevators and a large building complex.

When the dogs return to the Guide Dogs for the Blind, formal training begins under the supervision of a licensed instructor. The initial steps in the training program involve teaching basic obedience commands such as "come," "sit," and "fetch." The dog then must learn to work in a harness and master the commands "forward," "left," and "right." After five to six workouts, the dog is ready to advance to a residential area in San Rafael. Here the instructor teaches the dog to stop for curbs, and to make left and right turns. The instructor encourages the dog by positive reinforcement, praising the dog whenever it aims to please. After an initial period in a residential area, they move to a more heavily traveled area in central San Rafael. Here the dogs learn to cross streets, work on obstructions, and pay attention to moving traffic. They work in stores, buildings, elevators, and stairways. The dog then advances to training in the downtown area of San Francisco, where the animal must manifest initiative and responsibility to get around safely. The instructor is blindfolded while working with the dog. If the team passes this test, the dog is ready to be placed with a blind master.

The dogs, of course, learn when to stop and go at stoplights by the traffic movements, since they are unable to distinguish between red and green lights. I learned this one time in downtown Seattle when a blind man and his dog were waiting. The light was green, but there were no pedestrians and no cars. When I offered my assistance, he informed me of this problem.

The blind master comes to San Rafael for four weeks to receive instruction on how to handle and care for the dog. Any blind man or woman who is physically and temperamentally suited to use a guide dog is eligible. As of 1979, the Guide Dogs for the Blind had enrolled about 3,500 sightless persons. Although it costs approximately 5,000 dollars to produce each man-dog team, no charge is made for this service. The blind person who qualifies must need the dog to help achieve economic or social independence. Although the blind person is given custody of the dog, the animal continues to be owned by Guide Dogs for the Blind, Inc., so that the school has some control over the treatment of the dog. The person must sign a contract in which he or she promises to care for the dog properly, treat it kindly, and use it only as a guide.

More information may be obtained by writing to:

Guide Dogs for the Blind, Inc.
Box 1200
San Rafael, California, 94902

SEEING EYE DOG PROGRAM

This program celebrated its 50th anniversary in 1979. Using about 30 breeds of dogs, they have placed about 7,500 animals. The current placement rate is 200 per year in both the United States and Canada. They are now using chiefly Labrador retrievers, golden retrievers, and German shepherds. They have their own breeding programs for Labrador retrievers, both the black and the yellow, and the German shepherds.

At six to eight weeks of age, they place the dogs with 4-H students for one year. Then the pups are returned and trained for about 3 months before the blind person is brought in for a month of training with his or her dog. A modest fee of 150 dollars is requested, and the dog then becomes legally the property of the blind person. Any replacement dog is 50 dollars. This private, nonprofit organization can be contacted at:

Seeing Eye Dog Program
Washington Valley Road
Morristown, N.J. 07960

GUIDING EYES FOR THE BLIND

Guiding Eyes for the Blind is a nonprofit organization dedicated to providing independent mobility to qualified blind persons. The organization breeds its own animals, principally German shepherds and retrievers. After weaning, the dogs are placed with 4-H students for one year and then returned for a three- to five-month training period. Anyone in the United States is eligible to apply for an animal. They request a fee of 150 dollars for both the animal and for a 26-day instruction class for the owner. The address for this organization is:

Guiding Eyes for the Blind, Inc.
106 East 41st St.
New York, N.Y. 10017

GUIDE DOG FOUNDATION FOR THE BLIND

Labrador and golden retrievers are used by this foundation, which breeds many of its own dogs. "Puppy walkers" care for the animals for about one year. These include the 4-H clubs, the Boy-Girl Scouts, and some Lions Clubs. Dogs are placed throughout the world, including Canada, the United States, South America, Japan, and Israel. Anyone between the ages of 18 and 60 is eligible to apply. They have a flexible training program for their animals. They attempt to match the dog with the blind prospective owner. Their address is:

Guide Dog Foundation for the Blind
109-19 72nd Ave.
Forest Hills, N.Y. 11375

PILOT DOGS, INCORPORATED

This organization, begun in 1950, places dogs with the blind in the United States and also in some foreign countries. It utilizes boxers, German shepherds, Doberman pinchers, Labrador retrievers, and Vizslas. In addition to a small breeding program to provide dogs of the right temperament and size, they also accept gifts from private individuals and organizations. After a selection process, the dogs are placed with FFA and 4-H students, where they are raised in homes until one year of age. They then enter a training program of two to four months, depending on the animal's progress. Blind masters are invited for a four-weeks' training program, and then dogs are turned over to them if the dog and master are successful in adapting to one another. The dogs are owned by the blind person, although Pilot Dogs, Inc. provides some follow-up. The organization is nonprofit, providing the room and board, training program, and round-trip ticket at no cost to all of their clients. Their address is:

Pilot Dogs, Inc.
625 West Town
Columbus, OH 43215

Hearing Handicapped

AMERICAN HUMANE ASSOCIATION

The hearing dog program as now constituted had its origin in Minnesota early in 1976. When a dog belonging to a hearing-impaired resident who had trained it to respond to household sounds died, the owner immediately contacted the local television station, which directed her to the Society for the Prevention of Cruelty to Animals (SPCA). Since neither they nor anyone else had a hearing dog program, the SPCA hired an expert dog trainer who experimentally trained six dogs to serve the hearing impaired. The resulting success and publicity pointed to a need for such animals, but it was a program far greater than the Minnesota SPCA could handle. At that point, the program was turned over to the nationally based American Humane Association in Colorado.

Since 1976, AHA has trained over 100 dogs. They have employed an expert as a hearing dog placement counselor in the Englewood, Colorado, Training Program. At the present time, up to five dogs are placed each month by Laura Rhea, the resident counselor, who has an assistant with a hearing impairment. The dogs selected are mixed breeds from the Denver shelter, usually six months to one year old and of varying sizes. Before training, a veterinarian performs a thorough physical examination, and the dogs are neutered. The training program involves teaching the dogs to respond to burglar and smoke alarms and unfamiliar noises. Depending on the needs of the hearing-impaired person, they may also be trained to recognize the telephone, door bell, bell from a teletype/typewriter, emergency vehicles, or the cry of a child. Some are also trained to retrieve objects that are dropped by owners who cannot hear them fall. The cost for training is in excess of 2,000 dollars per dog. The recipient of one of these animals must be severely or profoundly deaf and have no other reasonable means of assistance.

Their address is:

The American Humane Association
Hearing Dog Program
5351 South Roslyn Street
Englewood, Colorado 80111

SAN FRANCISCO SPCA

The Hearing Dog Program selects dogs from the dog pound and trains and places them at no charge with people in the area who are hearing impaired. They emphasize careful follow-up after placement.

Their address is:

San Francisco SPCA
2500 16th Street
San Francisco, CA 94103

Physically Handicapped

Help for the disabled has been given by a group who formed a handi-persons or handi-dog program in the Southwest. The owners are themselves taught to train their dogs. They learn the beginning exercises of regular dog training and then add to them signals for picking up dropped objects, carrying things, barking on command, fetching newspapers and other items. The students in this program are also taught the American Kennel Club Obedience Competition Guidelines so that they can compete in dog obedience trials. The AKC has changed some of its rules to accommodate the disabled. This program has had a salutary effect on many people, for they take great pride in their ability to manage their dogs. One person, so debilitated by muscular dystrophy that he had effective motion only in his wrists, learned to control his dog and entered competition at the Obedience Club fun matches. He often won ribbons for his accomplishments. Every year since 1974, this handi-dog program has offered courses for the disabled and senior citizens, as well as a course for the hard of hearing.

An example of the significance of handi-dogs occurred with a little brown poodle owned by an elderly lady who was paralyzed from a stroke and lived alone. One evening she fell in her bedroom and lay unconscious on the floor, there being exposed to a cold draft from the open patio door. The dog had been trained to bark as a signal for help, and in this case barked for an hour until neighbors were aroused to investigate. The physician said without a doubt the dog had saved the woman's life (Gaines Dog Research Center, and published in *Today's Animal Health*).

CANINE COMPANIONS FOR INDEPENDENCE

This nonprofit corporation trains dogs to facilitate the independent living skills of the disabled community. The service dog is individually trained to the requirements of the physically disabled participant. The participant trains the dog with the help of a trainer from the corporation and later attends a public dog training class.

Their address is:

Canine Companions for Independence
P.O. Box 446
Santa Rosa, California 95402
(707) 528-0830

YOUNG ANIMAL SELECTION

Puppy

Since some older people have a great interest in young dogs, and often they have sufficient time to spend with the animal to train it, suggested procedures for selecting a puppy are included. It is important to note that the behavioral patterns of a dog are formed early in its development (Scott, 1962; Scott and Fuller, 1950, 1965; Pfaffenberger et al., 1976; Fox, 1965, 1971a, b, 1972, 1974, 1976, 1978; Whitney, 1971). Therefore, the owner should be knowledgeable about how to select and handle a young dog before the puppy is set in its ways, so as to prevent many of the problems that may emerge.

Numerous publications describe selection techniques. The following suggestions (Campbell, 1972; Vollmer, 1977, 1978) apply to an animal that is seven to sixteen weeks old. The objectives are to measure the dog's attachment to people (primary socialization) and its tolerance to authority (secondary socialization).

PRIMARY SOCIALIZATION

You can immediately eliminate from consideration any pup that does not approach you. Of those that approach, you then select from the pups those that you coax to you. Primary socialization really begins at about three weeks of age and requires daily physical contact of a nonthreatening type.

SECONDARY SOCIALIZATION

Elevation Test   This test is performed to determine the pup's tolerance for being in a raised position. Place both hands under the puppy's four legs and raise it with the muzzle towards you to a level just above your head for about half a minute. If the pup struggles, you raise your voice and shake it gently but firmly. If it settles down, you respond with a calm, soft voice. This is repeated three times, and if the pup does not manifest a calm response, it should be eliminated.

Inversion Test   This is done immediately after the elevation test. Holding the animal, rotate it on its back and hold it in this position for 30 seconds. Repeat this procedure three times in the manner of the elevation test. With gentle restraint and quiet reassurance, the animal should cease struggling.

Prone Test   Immediately following the inversion test, place the animal on the floor on its side, where it must lie quietly for 60 seconds. Grasp the scruff of the neck with one hand and use the free hand to quiet the struggle. In this procedure, stroke the pup's groin area; it should raise its hind leg. The free hand is also used to test the tolerance of facial manipulation by delivering moderate pressure to the muzzle.

Approach Test   In this final test, release the pup from the prone position. As soon as it arises, it should approach and seek body contact. If the pup does this, it should be petted and given words of encouragement. Then the person should walk away while encouraging the pup to follow. If the pup enthusiastically responds and has passed the other tests, this is probably a pup worthy of ownership.

These tests enable the prospective puppy owner to determine if the dog will accept a low-ranking position within the human "pack" as a companion animal. Eventually, such selection procedures may be evaluated and recommended for a variety of animal species. A more extensive version of this test that includes a scoring system, along with a review of literature on the subject, has been prepared by Melissa Bartlett (1979). She recommends testing during the seventh week of age.

Kitten

Cats should be obtained by 6 to 8 weeks of age and taught to play when young. It is well to choose kittens from a friendly mother and to select neither the most shy nor the most aggressive kitten. Some of the temperament traits listed on the adult cat profile are appropriate. Particularly, a kitten can be judged on the degree to which it actively seeks affection from people. Does it purr, meow, and approach people, or does it display hostile behavior when handled or approached? Is it adventurous, or does it act shy and cower? Is it playful or aloof? The usual criteria of good health, attractiveness, hair length, and propensity for indoor or outdoor living also have to be examined.

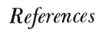

References

REFERENCES

Adler, W. H. (1974). An "autoimmune" theory of aging. In M. Rockenstein, M. L. Sussman, and J. Chesky, eds., *Theoretical Aspects of Aging.* New York: Academic Press.

—— (1975). Aging and the immune function. *Biol Sci.* 25:652-657.

Ahrens, E. H. (1979). Dietary fats and coronary heart disease: Unfinished business. *Lancet* 2: 1345-1348.

Ahuja, M. R., and F. Anders (1977). Cancer as a problem of gene regulation. In R. C. Gallo, ed. *Recent Advances in Cancer Research: Cell Biology, Molecular Biology and Tumor Virology.* Cleveland CRC Press.

Albanese, A. A. (1978). Calcium nutrition in the elderly. *Postgrad. Med.* 63(3): 167-172.

Almy, T. P. (1976). The role of fiber in the diet. In M. Winick, ed., *Nutrition and Aging.* New York: John Wiley and Sons.

Anderson, S., and W. H. Garritt (1966). The effect of a person on cardiac and motor responsivity to shock in dogs. *Conditioned Reflex* 1:181-189.

Andras, G. L., and W. R. Hazzard (1979). Plasma lipid, lipoproteins and lecithin: Cholesterol acyltransferase (LCAT). In D. M. Bowden, ed., *Aging in Nonhuman Primates.* New York: Van Nostrand Reinhold.

Andres, R., and J. D. Tobin (1977). In C. E. Finch and L. Hayflick, eds., *The Biology of Aging.* New York: Van Nostrand Reinhold.

Animal Humane Society of Hennepin Co. (1974). Pets by prescription. *Fact Sheet* Feb. 1.

Applewhite, T. H. (1979). Statistical "correlations" relating trans-fats to cancer: A commentary. *Fed. Proc.* 38:2435.

Arkow, P. S. (1973). Small animal lending library. *Animal Shelter Shoptalk* 21(12):2-3, 12.

193

—— (1976). A review of sources for pet therapy programs. *Humane Society of the Pikes Peak Region.* June.

—— (1977). Pet therapy, a study of the use of companion animals in selected therapies. *Humane Society of the Pikes Peak Region.*

Armstrong, M. L., and M. B. Megan (1972). Lipid depletion in atheromatous coronary arteries in rhesus monkeys after regression diets. *Circ. Res.* 30:675-680.

Armstrong, M. L., E. D. Warner, and W. E. Connor (1970). Regression of coronary atheromatosis in rhesus monkeys. *Circ. Res.* 27:59-67.

Asimov, I. (1965). The slowly moving finger. In *Of Time and Space and Other Things.* New York: Lancer Books.

Aslan, A., A. Vrabiescu, C. Domilescu, L. Campeanu, M. Costiniu, and S. Stanescu (1965). Long-term treatment with procaine (Gerovital H3) in albino rats. *J. Gerontol.* 20:1-8.

Baba, N., J. J. Quattrochi, P. B. Baker, and C. F. Mueller (1979). Cardiac and coronary pathology. In D. M. Bowden, ed., *Aging in Nonhuman Primates.* New York: Van Nostrand Reinhold.

Bailar, J. C. (1979). Dietary fat and cancer trends—a further critique. *Fed. Proc.* 38:2435-2436.

Baisley, M., M. F. Brink, and E. W. Speckman (1971). Nutrition in disease and stress. *Geriatrics* 26:87-93.

Balogh, K., and K. Lelkes (1961). The tongue in old age. *Gerontology* 3 Suppl.: 38-54.

Barloy, J. J. (1974). *Man and Animals, 100 Centuries of Friendship.* Translated by Henry Fox. New York: Gordon and Cremonsi.

Bartlett, M. (1979). A novice looks at puppy aptitude testing. *Purebred Dogs AKC Gazette* March:31-42.

Barzel, V. S. (1970). *Osteoporosis.* New York: Grune and Stratton.

—— (1978). Common metabolic disorders of the skeleton in aging. In W. Reichel, ed., *Clinical Aspects of Aging.* Baltimore: Williams and Wilkins.

Bass, L. (1977). More fiber—less constipation. *Am. J. Nurs.* 77:254-255.

Bath, M., A. Krook, G. Sandquist, and K. Stantze (1976). *Is the Dog Needed? A Study of the Dog's Social Importance to Man.* Thesis: School of Social Studies, University of Göteborg. Göteborg, Sweden.

Bazzarre, T. L. (1978). Aging and nutrition education. *Ed. Gerontol.* 3:149-163.

Beare-Rogers, J. L., L. M. Gray, and R. Hollywood (1979). The linoleic acid and trans fatty acids of margarines. *Am. J. Clin. Nutr.* 32:1805-1809.

Beck, A. (1975). The public health implications of urban dogs. *Am. J. Public Health* 65:1315-1318.

Beeson, P. B. (1979). Training doctors to care for old people. *Ann. Int. Med.* 90: 262-263.

Behnke, J. A., C. E. Finch, and G. B. Moment, eds. (1978). *The Biology of Aging.* New York: Plenum Press.

Belt, Ed. (1952) Leonardo da Vinci's study of the aging process. *Geriatrics* 7:205-210.

Benson, H., T. Dryer, and H. Hartley (1978). Decreased oxygen consumption during exercise with elicitation of the relaxation response. *J. Human Stress* 4(2):38-42.

Berg, B., and H. S. Simms (1960a). Nutrition and longevity in the rat. I. Food intake in relation to size, health and fertility. *J. Nutr.* 71:242-255.

—— (1960b). Nutrition and longevity in the rat. II. Longevity and onset of disease with different levels of food intake. *J. Nutr.* 71:255-263.

Bevan, W. (1972). On growing old in America. *Science* 177:839.

Bierman, E. L. (1976). Obesity, carbohydrate and lipid interactions in the elderly. In M. Winick, ed., *Nutrition and Aging.* New York: John Wiley and Sons.

Biorck, G., W. Overbeck, and C. Gronvall (1954). Coronarkrankheit und herzinfarkt in Malmo. Ein beitrag zur geographischen pathologie der coronarkrankheit. *Cardiologia* 25:232.

Birenbaum, A., M. Aronson, and S. Seiffer (1979). Training medical students to appreciate special problems of the elderly. *The Gerontologist* 19:575-579.

Bjorksten, J. (1968). The cross linkage theory of aging. *J. Am. Gerontol. Soc.* 16:408-427.

—— (1974). Cross linkage and the aging process. In M. Rockstein, M. Sussman, and J. Chesky, eds., *Theoretical Aspects of Aging.* New York: Academic Press.

Blankenhorn, D. H. (1977). Studies of regression/progression of atherosclerosis in man. In G. W. Manning and M. D. Haust, eds., *Atherosclerosis. Adv. Exp. Med. Biol.* 82:453-458. New York: Plenum Press.

Blankwater, M. J. (1978). *Ageing and the Humoral Immune Response in Mice.* Rijswijk, Netherlands: Institute of Experimental Gerontology.

Blount, W. P. (1961). Turkey X disease. *Turkeys (J. Br. Turkey Fed.)* 9:52.

Blumenthal, H. T. (1978). Aging: Biologic or pathologic. *Hosp. Pract.* 13(4): 127-137.

Bourne, G. H. (1956). Physiological and cellular aspects of aging. *Nature* 178: 839-840.

Boutwell, R. K. (1964). Some biological aspects of skin carcinogenesis. *Prog. Exp. Tumor Res.* 4:207-250.

—— (1974). The function and mechanism of promotors of carcinogenesis. *CRC Critical Reviews in Toxicology,* January.

Bowden, D. M., ed. (1979). *Aging in Nonhuman Primates.* New York: Van Nostrand Reinhold.

Bowden, D. M., and M. L. Jones. (1979). Aging research in nonhuman primates. In D. M. Bowden, ed., *Aging in Nonhuman Primates.* New York: Van Nostrand Reinhold.

Bowden, D. M., C. Teets, S. Witkin, and D. M. Young (1979). Long bone calcification and morphology. In D. M. Bowden, ed., *Aging in Nonhuman Primates.* New York: Van Nostrand Reinhold.

Brace, C. L. (1962). Physique, physiology, and behavior: An attempt to analyse a part of their roles in the canine biogram. Unpublished doctoral dissertation, Harvard University.

Brash, D. E., and R. W. Hart (1978). Molecular biology of aging. In J. A. Behnke, C. E. Finch, and G. B. Moment, eds., *The Biology of Aging.* New York: Plenum Press.

Brickel, C. M. (1979). The therapeutic roles of cat mascots with a hospital-based geriatric population: A staff survey. *Gerontologist* 19:368-372.

Brin, M., and J. C. Bauernfiend (1978). Vitamin needs of the elderly. *Postgrad Med.* 63(3):155-163.

Brodie, J. D. (1979). The role of the veterinarian. *Group for the Study of the Human/Companion Animal Bond Newsletter.* 1(1):5-13.

Brody, H. (1976). An examination of the cerebral cortex and brain stem aging.

In R. D. Terry and S. Gersbon, eds., *Neurobiology of Aging.* New York: Raven Press.

Brody, H., and N. Vijayashankar (1977). Anatomical changes in the nervous system. In C. E. Finch and L. Hayflick, eds., *Handbook of the Biology of Aging.* New York: Van Nostrand Reinhold.

Brody, S. (1945). *Bioenergetics and Growth.* New York: Reinhold Publishing Co.

Brown, W. H., L. Pearce, and C. M. Van Allen (1926). Organ weights of normal rabbits—second paper. *J. Exp. Med.* 43:733-741.

Brunzell, J. D., A. Chait, and E. L. Bierman (1978). Pathophysiology of lipoprotein transport. *Metabolism* 27:1109-1127.

Buckwald, H., R. B. Moore, and R. L. Varco (1975). The partial ileal bypass operation in treatment of hyperlipidemias. In D. Kritchevsky, R. Paoletti, and W. L. Holmes, eds., *Lipids, Lipoproteins and Drugs. Adv. Exp. Med. Biol.* 63:221-230. New York: Plenum Press.

Bullamore, J. R., J. C. Gallagher, R. Wilkinson, B. E. C. Nordin, and D. H. Marshall (1970). Effect of age on calcium absorption. *Lancet* 2:535-537.

Burkitt, D. P., A. R. Walker, and N. S. Painter (1972). Effect of dietary fibre on stools and transit times and its role in the causation of disease. *Lancet* 2:1408-1413.

Burnet, F. M. (1974). *Intrinsic Mutagenesis: A Genetic Approach to Aging.* New York: John Wiley and Sons.

Burnside, I. M. (1976). Mental health in the aged: The nurse's perspective. In R. H. Davis, ed., *Aging: Prospects and Issues.* Los Angeles: The University of Southern California Press.

—— (1976). Realities of working with the aged. In R. H. Davis, ed., *Aging: Prospects and Issues.* Los Angeles: The University of Southern California Press.

Busch, H. (1979). The complexity of the cancer problem. *Fed. Proc.* 38:94-96.

Busse, E. W. (1978). How mind, body, and environment influence nutrition in the elderly. *Postgrad. Med.* 63(3):118-128.

Bustad, L. K. (1960). *Physiological Responses of Mice to Low Levels of Irradiation.* Seattle, University of Washington, Ph.D. Thesis.

—— (1966). Pigs in the laboratory. *Sci. Am.* 214(6):94-100.

—— (1970). The experimental subject—a choice, not an echo. *Perspect. Biol. Med.* 14(1):1-10.

—— (1973). The problem and paradox that is cancer. In C. L. Sanders, R. H. Busch, J. E. Ballou, and D. D. Mahlum, eds., *Radionuclide Carcinogenesis.* Office of Information Services, U. S. Atomic Energy Commission, Washington, DC.

—— (1976a). Dose and dose rate problems in radiation tumorigenesis. In G. Walinder, ed., *Symposium on Tumorigenic and Genetic Effects of Radiation.* Stockholm: National Swedish Environment Protection Board. 695:107-128.

—— (1976b). Pets-for-people therapy. *West. Vet.* 14(2):28-31.

—— (1976c). A report of your peripatetic dean. *West. Vet.* 14(2):35-36.

—— (1978a). Pets for people-therapy. *Today's Animal Health* 9(5):9-10.

—— (1978b). The peripatetic dean: Bethel visit. *West. Vet.* 16(3):2.

—— (1979a). How animals make people human and humane. *Proceedings of Second Canadian Symposium on Pets and Society.* Toronto, Ontario. Dr. Ballards Pet Food Div. Standard Brands Food Co.

—— (1979b). Profiling animals for therapy. *West. Vet.* 17(1):2.

—— (1979c). Current challenges in comparative medicine. John Gunion Rutherford Memorial Lecture, University of Saskatchewan, Saskatoon, Saskatchewan, Canada, March 26.

—— (1979d). People-pet partnership. *West. Vet.* 17(3):2-4.

Bustad, L. K., N. M. Gates, A. Ross, and L. D. Carlson (1965). Effects of prolonged low-level irradiation of mice. *Rad. Res.* 25:318-330.

Bustad, L. K., J. R. Gorham, G. A. Hegreberg, and G. A. Padgett (1976). Comparative medicine: Progress and prospects. *J. Am. Vet. Med. Assoc.* 169:90-105.

Bustad, L. K., and L. H. Hines (1980). Human-companion animal bond and the curriculum. In B. Fogel, ed., *Proc. Br. Small Anim. Vet. Assoc. Meeting on the Human/Companion Animal Bond.* London, England (in press).

Bustad, L. K., and R. O. McClellan, eds. (1966). *Swine in Biomedical Research.* Seattle, WA: Frayn Printing Co.

Bustad, L. K., L. S. Rosenblatt, and J. L. Palotay (1968). The use of miniature swine in gerontological research. In *The Laboratory Animal in Gerontological Research.* Washington, DC: National Academy of Science Publication 1591.

Bustad, L. K., D. E. Warner, and H. A. Kornberg (1958). Effect of stable iodine on uptake of radioiodine in sheep. *Am. J. Vet. Res.* 19:893-894.

Butler, R. N. (1975). *Why Survive? Being Old in America.* New York: Harper and Row.

Butler, R. N., and B. Gastel (1979). Aging and cancer management. Part II: Research perspectives. *CA.* 29:333-340.

Campbell, M. J., A. J. McComas, and F. J. Petito (1973). Physiological changes in ageing muscles. *J. Neurol. Neurosurg. Psychiatry* 36:174-182.

Campbell, W. E. (1972) A behavior test for puppy selection. *Mod. Vet. Pract.* December: 29-33.

Canby, T. Y. (1979). The search for the first Americans. *Natl. Geograph.* 156(3): 348.

Carding, A. (1975). The growth of pet populations in Western Europe and the implication for dog control in Great Britain. In R. S. Anderson, ed., *Pet Animals and Society.* Baltimore: Williams and Wilkins.

Carlson, H. E., J. C. Gillin, P. Gordon, and F. Snyder (1972). Absence of sleep-related growth hormone peaks in aged normal subjects and in acromegaly. *J. Clin. Endocrinol. Metab.* 34:1102-1105.

Carlson, L. A. and B. Kolmodin-Hedman (1977). Decrease in alpha-lipoprotein cholesterol in men after cessation of exposure to chlorinated hydrocarbon pesticides. *Acta Med. Scand.* 201:375-376.

Carlson, L. D., W. J. Scheyer, and B. H. Jackson (1957). The combined effects of ionizing radiation and low temperature on the metabolism, longevity, and soft tissues of the white rat. I. Metabolism and longevity. *Radiation Res.* 7:190-197.

Carrel, A. (1935). *Man the Unknown.* New York: Harper.

Carroll, K. K. (1975). Experimental evidence of dietary factors and hormone-dependent cancers. *Cancer Res.* 35:3374-3383.

Carroll, K. K., and H. T. Khor (1971). Effects of level and type of dietary fat on incidence of mammary tumors induced in female Sprague-Dawley rats by 7,12 dimethylbenzanthracene. *Lipids* 6:415-420.

Castelli, W. P., J. T. Doyle, T. Gordon, C. G. Hames, M. C. Hjortland, S. B. Hulley, A. Kagan, and W. Zukel (1977). HDL cholesterol and other lipids in coronary heart disease: The cooperative lipoprotein phenotyping study. *Circulation* 55:767-772.

Cattell, R. B., and B. Korth (1973). The isolation of temperament dimensions in dogs. *Behav. Biol.* 9:15-30. Abstract 179R.

Child, C. M. (1915). *Senescence and Rejuvenescence.* Chicago: University of Chicago Press, 11:481.

Clark, R. L., and F. J. Rauscher (1977). Cancer: A search for both cures and causes. *Washington Post.* Washington, DC, May 12.

Clarke, M., and L. M. Wakefield (1975). Food choices of institutionalized vs. independent-living elderly. *J. Am. Dietetic Assoc.* 66:600-604.

Clarkson, T. B., J. S. King, H. B. Lofland Jr., M. A. Feldner, and B. C. Bullock (1973). Characteristics and composition of diet-aggravated atherosclerotic plaques during "regression." *J. Mol. Pathol.* 19:267-283.

Clarkson, T. B., N. D. Lehner, W. D. Wagner, R. W. St. Clair, M. G. Bond, and B. C. Bullock (1979). A study of atherosclerosis regression in Macaca mulatta. *Exp. Mol. Pathol.* 30:360-385.

Clarkson, T. B., R. W. Prichard, B. C. Bullock, R. W. St. Clair, N. D. M. Lehner, D. C. Jones, W. D. Wagner, and L. L. Rudel (1976). Pathogenesis of atherosclerosis; some advances from using animal models. *Exp. Mol. Pathol.* 24: 264-286.

Clarkson, T. B., R. W. Prichard, M. G. Netsky, and H. B. Lofland (1959). Atherosclerosis in pigeons. Its spontaneous occurrence and resemblance in human atherosclerosis. *Arch. Pathol.* 68:143-147.

Clawson, B. J. (1941). Incidence of types of heart disease among 30,265 autopsies with special reference to age and sex. *Am. Heart J.* 22:607-624.

Clemens, J. A., R. W. Fuller, and N. V. Owen (1978). Some neuroendocrine aspects of aging. In C. E. Finch, D. E. Potter, and A. D. Kenny, eds., *Parkinson's Disease II. Aging and Neuroendocrine Relationships.* New York: Plenum Press.

Cohen, B. J. (1979). Dietary factors affecting rats used in aging research. *J. Gerontol.* 34:803-807.

Collins, K. J., C. Dore, A. N. Exton-Smith, R. H. Fox, I. C. MacDonald, and P. M. Woodward (1977). Accidental hypothermia and impaired temperature homeostasis in the elderly. *Br. Med. J.* 1:353-356.

Comfort, A. (1956). *The Biology of Senescence.* London: Routeledge and Kegan Paul Ltd.

—— (1964). *Aging, the Biology of Senescence.* New York: Holt, Rhinehart and Winston.

—— (1971). Why not cancer and aging research? *Med. Opinion* 7(4):10-11.

—— (1979). *The Biology of Senescence.* 3rd ed. New York: Elsevier North-Holland, Inc.

Committee on Food Protection, Food and Nutrition Board, National Research Council (1973). *Toxicants Occurring Naturally in Foods,* 2nd ed. Washington, DC: National Academy of Sciences.

Connor, W. E., and S. L. Connor (1972). The key role of nutritional factors in the prevention of coronary heart disease. *Prev. Med.* 1:49-83.

Cooper, J. E. (1976). Pets in hospitals. *Br. Med. J.* 1:698-700.

Corson, S. A., and E. O'L. Corson (1979). Pets as mediators of therapy in custodial institutions and the aged. In J. H. Masserman, ed., *Current Psychiatric Therapies.* Vol. 18. New York: Grune and Stratton.

Corson, S. A., E. O'L. Corson, and P. H. Gwynne (1975). Pet-facilitated psychotherapy. In R. S. Anderson, ed., *Pet Animals and Society.* Baltimore: Williams and Wilkins.

Corson, S. A., E. O'L. Corson, P. H. Gwynne, and L. E. Arnold (1977). Pet dogs as nonverbal communication links in hospital psychiatry. *Compr. Psychiatry* 18: 61-72.

Cotzias, G. C., S. T. Miller, L. C. Tang, P. S. Papavasiliou, and Y. Y. Wang (1977). Levodopa, fertility, and longevity. *Science* 196:549-551.

Creel, H. L. (1976). *Cooking for One is Fun.* New York: Quadrangle/The New York Times Book Co.

Culliton, B. J. (1978). Toxic substances legislation: How well are laws being implemented? *Science* 201:1198-1199.

Cummings, J. H. (1978). Nutritional implications of dietary fiber. *Am. J. Clin. Nutr.* 31 Oct.:521-529.

Cutler, R. G. (1978). Evolutionary biology of senescence. In J. A. Behnke, C. E. Finch, and G. B. Moment, eds., *The Biology of Aging.* New York: Plenum Press.

Dauod, A. S., J. Jarmolych, J. M. Augustyn, K. E. Fritz, J. K. Singh, and K. T. Lee (1976). Regression of advanced atherosclerosis in swine. *Arch. Pathol. Lab. Med.* 100:372-379.

Davies, P. (1978). Loss of choline acetyltransferase activity in normal aging and in senile dementia. In C. E. Finch, D. E. Potter, and A. D. Kenny, eds., *Parkinson's Disease II. Aging and Neuroendocrine Relationships.* New York: Plenum Press.

Davis, D. L., and B. H. Magee (1979). Cancer and industrial chemical production. *Science* 206:1356, 1358.

Davis, S. J. M., and F. R. Valla (1978). Evidence for domestication of the dog 12000 years ago in the Natufian of Israel. *Nature* 276:608-610.

Dement, W. C. (1972). *Some Must Watch While Some Must Sleep.* Stanford, CA: Stanford Alumni Association.

Deming, Q. B. (1975). Hypertension and other risk factors. *Adv. Exp. Med. Biol.* 63:287-303.

Denckla, W. D. (1975). A time to die. *Life Sciences* 16:31-44.

Denckla, W. D. (1977). Systems analysis of possible mechanisms of mammalian aging. *Mechanisms of Aging and Development* 6:143-152.

DePalma, R. G., E. M. Bellon, L. Klein, S. Koletsky, and W. Insull, Jr. (1977). Approaches to evaluating regression of experimental atherosclerosis. *Adv. Exp. Med. Biol.* 82:459-470.

DePalma, R. G., W. Insull, Jr., E. M. Bellon, W. T. Roth, and A. V. Robinson (1972). Animal models for the study of progression and regression of atherosclerosis. *Surgery* 72:268-278.

Detweiler, D. K. (1966). Swine in comparative cardiovascular research. In L. K. Bustad and R. O. McClellan, eds., *Swine in Biomedical Research.* Seattle: Frayn Printing.

Devesa, S. S., and D. T. Silverman (1978). Cancer incidence and mortality trends in the United States: (1935-74). *J. Natl. Cancer Inst.* 60:545-571

DeVries, N. A. (1968). *Report on Jogging and Exercise for Older Adults.* Washington, DC: U.S. Administration on Aging. U.S. Department of Health, Education, and Welfare.

Dhar, N. R. (1926). Old age and death from a chemical point of view. *J. Physical Chem.* 30:378-382.

—— (1930). Influence of aging on inorganic hydrophile colloids, cells and colloids in the animal body. *J. Physical Chem.* 34:549-553.

Dill, D. B., S. M. Horvath, and F. N. Craig (1958). Responses to exercise as related to age. *J. Appl. Physiol.* 12:195-196.

Dutton, H. J. (1974). Analysis and monitoring of trans-isomerization by IR attenuated total reflectance spectrophotometry. *Am. Oil Chem. Soc.* 51:407-409.

Eckstein, R. W. (1957). Effect of exercise and coronary artery narrowing on coronary collateral circulation. *Circ. Res.* 5:230-235.

Edds, G. T. (1973). Acute aflatoxicosis: A review. *J. Am. Vet. Med. Assoc.* 162: 304-309.

Ellermann, V., and O. Bang (1908). Experimentelle leukamie bei huhnern. *Zentralbl. Bakteriol.* 46:595-609.

Ender, F., G. Havre, A. Hedgebostad, N. Koppang, R. Madsen, and L. Ceh (1964). Isolation and identification of a hepatotoxic factor in herring meal produced from sodium nitrite preserved herring. *Naturwissenschaften* 51:637-638.

Engelhardt, W. V. (1966). Swine cardiovascular physiology—a review. In L. K. Bustad and R. O. McClellan, eds., *Swine in Biomedical Research.* Seattle: Frayn Printing.

Enig, M. G., R. J. Munn, and M. Keeney (1978). Dietary fat and cancer trends— a critique. *Fed. Proc.* 37:2215-2220.

—— (1979). Response. *Fed. Proc.* 38:2437-2439.

Ensminger, M. E. (1977). *The Complete Book of Dogs.* New York: A. S. Barnes.

Enstrom, J. E., and D. F. Austin (1978). Interpreting cancer survival rates. In P. H. Abelson, ed., *Health Care: Regulation, Economics, Ethics, Practice.* Washington, DC: American Association for the Advancement of Science.

Essex, M. (1979). Etiology of leukemia in outbred animal species. In G. P. Margison, ed., *Advances in Medical Oncology,* New York: Pergamon Press.

Essex, M., G. Todaro, and H. Zurhausen, eds. (1980). *Role of Viruses in Naturally Occurring Cancer.* Cold Spring Harbor, Long Island: Cold Spring Harbor Press.

Everitt, A. V. (1973). *The Hypothalamic-pituitary Control of Ageing and Age-Related Pathology.* Sydney: Pergamon Press.

Fallat, R. W., C. J. Clueck, R. Lutmer, and F. H. Mattson (1976). Short-term study of sucrose polyester, a nonabsorbable fat-like material, as a dietary agent for lowering plasma cholesterol. *Am. J. Clin. Nutr.* 29:1204-1215.

Fassett, D. W. (1973). Nitrates and nitrites. In *Toxicants Occurring Naturally in Foods.* 2nd ed. Washington, DC: National Academy of Sciences.

Feinberg, I. (1976). Functional implications of changes in sleep physiology with age. In R. D. Terry and S. Gershon, eds., *Neurobiology of Aging.* New York: Raven Press.

Feinberg, I., M. Braun, and R. L. Koresko (1969). Vertical eye-movement during REM sleep: Effects of age and electrode placement. *Psychophysiol.* 5:556-561.

Fernandes, G., E. J. Yunis, and R. A. Good (1976). Influence of diet on survival of mice. *Proc. Natl. Acad. Sci. USA* 73:1279-1283.

Fernandes, G., E. J. Yunis, M. Miranda, J. Smith, and R. A. Good (1978). Nutritional inhibition of genetically determined renal disease and autoimmunity with prolongation of life in kdkd mice. *Proc. Natl. Acad. Sci. USA* 75:2888-2892.

Finch, C. E. (1969). *Cellular Activities During Aging in Mammals.* Ph.D. Thesis, New York. The Rockefeller University.

—— (1973). Catecholamine metabolism on the brains of aging male mice. *Brain Res.* 52:261-276.

—— (1975). Neuroendocrinology of aging: A view of an emerging area. *BioScience* 25:645-650.

—— (1976). The regulation of physiological changes during mammalian aging. *Quart. Rev. Biol.* 51:49-83.

—— (1977). Neuroendocrine and autonomic aspects of aging. In C. E. Finch and L. Hayflick, eds., *Handbook of the Biology of Aging.* New York: Van Nostrand Reinhold.

—— (1978a). Age-related changes in brain catecholamines: A synopsis of findings in C57BL/6J mice and other rodent models. In C. E. Finch, D. E. Potter, and A. D. Kenny, eds., *Parkinson's Disease II. Aging and Neuroendocrine Relationships.* New York: Plenum Press.

—— (1978b). The brain and aging. In J. A. Behnke, C. E. Finch, and G. B. Moment, eds., *The Biology of Aging.* New York: Plenum Press.

—— (1979). Neuroendocrine mechanisms of aging. *Fed. Proc.* 38:178-183.

Finch, C. E., J. R. Foster, and A. E. Marsky (1969). Aging and regulation of cell activities. *J. Gen. Physiol.* 54:690-712.

Finch, C. E., and L. Hayflick (1977). *Handbook of the Biology of Aging.* New York: Van Nostrand Reinhold.

Finch, C. E., D. E. Potter, and A. D. Kenny, eds. (1978). *Parkinson's Disease II. Aging and Neuroendocrine Relationships.* New York: Plenum Press.

Fogle, B. (1979). Review and discussion of future plans. *Proceedings of Meeting of Group for the Study of Human/Companion Animal Bond.* Dundee, England; March 23-25.

Fox, H. (1933). Arteriosclerosis in lower mammals and birds: Its relation to the disease in man. In E. V. Cowdry, ed., *Arteriosclerosis.* New York: Macmillan.

Fox, M. W. (1965). *Canine Behavior.* Springfield, IL: Charles C. Thomas.

—— (1971a). *Integrative Development of Brain and Behavior in the Dog.* Chicago: The University of Chicago Press.

—— (1971b). *Behavior of Wolves, Dogs and Related Canids.* New York: Harper & Row.

—— (1972). *Understanding Your Dog.* New York: Coward, McCann and Geohegan.

—— (1974). *Concepts in Ethology: Animal and Human Behavior.* Minneapolis: University of Minnesota Press.

—— (1976). *Between Animal and Man.* New York: Coward, McCann and Geohegan.

—— (1978). *The Dog: Its Domestication and Behavior.* New York: Garland STPM Press.

Friedmann, E. (1979). Pet ownership and survival after coronary heart disease. *Proceedings of Second Canadian Symposium on Pets and Society.* Toronto, Ontario: Dr. Ballards Pet Food Div. Standard Brands Food.

Fritz, K. E., J. M. Augustyn, J. Jarmolych, A. S. Daoud, and K. T. Lee (1976). Regression of advanced atherosclerosis in swine. *Arch. Pathol. Lab. Med.* 100:380-385.

Froelicher, V. F. (1972). Animal studies of effect of chronic exercise of the heart and atherosclerosis: A review. *Am. Heart J.* 84:496-506.

Fuster, V., and E. J. Bowie (1978). The von Willebrand pig as a model for atherosclerosis research. *Thromb. Haemostas.* 39:322-327.

Gajdusek, D. C. (1974). Slow and latent viruses and the aging nervous system. In G. J. Malitta, ed., *Survey Report on the Aging Nervous System,* DHEW (NIH) 74-296. Washington DC: U.S. Government Printing Office.

Gaines Dog Research Center (1978). Dogs in a new role. *Gaines Progress,* Summer ed., pp. 1, 6-7.

Gallo, R. C., ed. (1977). *Recent Advances in Cancer Research: Cell Biology, Molecular Biology, and Tumor Virology.* Cleveland: CRC Press.

Gingrich, R. D., and J. C. Hoak (1979). Platelet-endothelial cell interactions. *Seminars in Hematology.* 16:208-220.

Glomset, J. A. (1979). Lecithin: Cholesterol acyltransferase. *Prog. Biochem. Pharmacol.* 15:41-66.

—— (1980). High density lipoproteins in human health and disease. *Adv. Intern. Med.* 25:91-116.

Goering, E. K. (1978). Counseling the owner of the terminal patient. Senior paper, Washington State University College of Veterinary Medicine.

Goldstein, S., and W. Reichel (1978). Physiological and biological aspects of aging. In W. Reichel, ed., *Clinical Aspects of Aging.* Baltimore: Williams and Wilkins.

Gonzalez, E. R. (1979). Exercise therapy "rediscovered" for diabetes, but what does it do? *J. Am. Med. Assoc.* 242:1591.

Goodwin, D. V. (1979). Sleep research: the chronological view. *Research Resources Reporter* 3(6). Bethesda, MD: National Institutes of Health.

Gordan, G. S., and C. Vaughan (1976). *Clinical Management of Osteoporoses.* Action, MA: Publishing Sciences Group.

Gordon, P. (1974). Free radicals and the aging process. In M. Rockstein, M. L. Sussman, and J. Chesky, eds., *Theoretical Aspects of Aging.* New York: Academic Press.

Gordon, T., W. P. Castelli, M. C. Hjortland, W. B. Kannel, and T. R. Dawber (1977a). High density lipoprotein as a protective factor against coronary heart disease: The Framingham study. *Am. J. Med.* 62:707-714.

—— (1977b). Diabetes, blood lipids and the role of obesity in coronary heart disease risk for women. The Framingham Study. *Ann. Intern. Med.* 87:393-397.

Gortner, W. A. (1975). Nutrition in the United States, 1900-1974. *Cancer Res.* 35:3246-3253.

Graham, S. (1837). *Treatise on Bread and Bread Making.* Boston: Light and Stearn.

Gregerman, R. I., and E. I. Bierman (1974). Aging and hormones. In R. H. Williams, ed., *Textbook of Endocrinology,* 5th ed. Philadelphia: W. B. Saunders.

Griesemer, R. A. (1979). *Risk of Cancer from Chemicals.* Presented at AVMA meeting, Seattle, July 25.

Gudbrandsen, C. O. (1961). The effect of physical exercise on cholesterol-induced atherosclerosis in rabbits. *Technical report 60-2.* Fort Wainwright, AK: Arctic Aeromedical Laboratory.

Gutmann, E. (1977). Muscle. In C. E. Finch and L. Hayflick, eds., *Handbook of the Biology of Aging.* New York, Van Nostrand Reinhold.

Hadlow, W. J. (1959). Scrapie and Kuru. *Lancet* 2:289-290.

Haenszel, W. (1961). Cancer mortality among the foreign-born in the United States. *J. Natl. Cancer Inst.* 26:37-132.

Hall, G. S., and C. E. Browne (1904). The cat and the child. *Pedagogical Seminary* 11:3-29.

Hall, R. L. (1977). Safe at the plate. *Nutr. Today* 12(6):6-9, 28-31.

Halliday, W. R. (1922). Animal pets in ancient Greece. *Discovery* 3:151-154.

Harman, D. (1956). A theory based on free radical and radiation chemistry. *J. Gerontol.* 11:298-299.

—— (1960). The free radical theory of aging: The effect of age on serum mercaptan levels. *J. Gerontol.* 15:38-40.

Harper, A. E. (1978). Recommended dietary allowances for the elderly. *Nutrition* 33(5):73-75, 79-80.

Hart, B. L. (1978). Feline behavior. *Feline Practice* 8:8-12.

Hay, R. J., and B. L. Strehler (1967). The limited growth span of cell strains isolated from the chick embryo. *Exp. Gerontol.* 2:123-135.

Hayflick, L. (1965). The limited *in vitro* lifetime of human diploid cell strains isolated from the chick embryo. *Exp. Cell Res.* 37:614-636.

—— (1970). Aging under glass. *Exp. Gerontol.* 5:291-303.

—— (1975). Current theories of biological aging. *Fed. Proc.* 34:9-13.

—— (1977). The cellular basis for biological aging. In C. E. Finch and L. Hayflick, eds., *Handbook of the Biology of Aging.* New York: Van Nostrand Reinhold.

—— (1980). The cell biology of human aging. *Sci. Am.* 242:58-65.

Hazzard, W. R. (1976). Aging and atherosclerosis: Interactions with diet, heredity, and associated risk factors. In M. Rockstein and M. L. Sussman, eds., *Nutrition, Longevity, and Aging.* New York: Academic Press.

—— (1979). Three views on geriatric medicine: 2: An American's ode to British geriatrics. *Age Ageing.* 8(3):141-143.

Hediger, H. (1965). Man as a social partner of animals and vice-versa. *Symp. Zool. Soc. Lond.* 14:291-300.

Hegsted, D. M. (1975a). Dietary standards. *J. Am. Dietetic Assoc.* 66:13-21.

—— (1975b). Dietary standards. *N. Engl. J. Med.* 292:915-917.

—— (1977). Food and fibre: Evidence from experimental animals. *Nutr. Rev.* 35(3):45-50.

Henkin, R. I., P. J. Schecter, W. T. Friedewald, D. L. Demets, and M. Raff (1976). A double blind study of the effects of zinc sulfate on taste and smell dysfunction. *Am. J. Med. Sci.* 272:285-299.

Hennekens, C. H., W. Willett, B. Rosner, D. S. Cole, and S. L. Mayrent (1979). Effects of beer, wine, and liquor in coronary deaths. *J. Am. Med. Assoc.* 242:1973-1974.

Herriot, J. (1977). *All Things Wise and Wonderful.* New York: St. Martin's Press.

Hesketh, B. (1978). The role of the dog in human development and mental health. Paper presented to the *Dog Seminar,* Hamilton, N. Zealand.

Higginson, J. and C. S. Muir (1979). Environmental carcinogenesis: Misconceptions and limitations to cancer control. *J. Natl. Cancer Inst.* 63:1291-1298.

Hill, M. J., J. S. Crowther, B. S. Drasar, G. Hawksworth, V. Aires, and R. E. O. Williams (1971). Bacteria and aetiology of cancer of large bowel. *Lancet* 1: 95-100.

Hill, M. J., B. S. Drasar, R. E. O. Williams, T. W. Meade, A. G. Cox, J. E. P. Simpson, and B. C. Morson (1975). Bile acids, bacteria and colon cancer. *Lancet* 1: 535-538.

Hines, D. M. (1976). *Tales of the Okanogans*. Fairfield, WA: Ye Galleon Press.

Hipsley, E. H. (1958). Coronary heart disease in Australia. *Nutr. Rev.* 16:129-131.

Hoffer, A. (1977). Supernutrition. In R. J. Williams and D. K. Kalita, eds., *A Physician's Handbook on Orthomolecular Medicine*. New York: Pergamon Press.

Hollander, C. F. (1978). Experimental gerontological research. *Ned. T. Geront.* 9:125-128.

Holloszy, J. O. (1971). Morphological and enzymatic adaptations to training—a review. In O. A. Larsen and R. O. Malmborg, eds., *Coronary Heart Disease and Physical Fitness*. Baltimore: University Park Press.

Holloway, W. D., C. Tasman-Jones, and S. P. Lee (1978). Digestion of certain fractions of dietary fiber in humans. *Am. J. Clin. Nutr.* 31:927-930.

Hopkins, G. A., and C. E. West (1976). Possible roles of dietary fats in carcinogenesis. *Life Sci.* 19:1103-1116.

Howard, C. F., Jr. (1973). Atherosclerosis in spontaneously diabetic monkeys. *Circulation* 48 (Suppl. IV):41.

—— (1975). Diabetes and lipid metabolism in nonhuman primates. In R. Paoletti and D. Kritchevsky, eds., *Adv. Lipid Res.*, Vol. 13. New York: Academic Press.

Howard, N., and S. Antilla (1979). What price safety? The "zero risk" debate. *Dun's Review* 114(3):48-57.

Huxley, T. H. (1888). *Science and Culture*. London: Macmillan.

Issenberg, P. (1976). Nitrite, nitrosamines, and cancer. *Fed. Proc.* 35:1322-1326.

Jarvik, L. F., A. Falek, F. J. Kallman, and I. Large (1960). Survival trends in a senescent twin population. *Am. J. Hum. Genet.* 12:170-179.

Jenkins, D. J. A., A. R. Leeds, C. Newton, and J. H. Cummings (1975). Effect of pectin, guargum, and wheat fibre on serum-cholesterol. *Lancet* 1:1116-1117.

Jernigan, J. (1973). Pet therapy brings happiness to the lonely. *Nat. Humane Rev.* Nov.:13.

Johnson, H. A., and S. Erner (1972). Neuron survival in the aging mouse. *Exp. Gerontol.* 7:111-117.

Jones, H. B. (1956). A special consideration of the aging process, disease and life expectancy. In J. H. Lawrence and C. A. Tobias, eds., *Adv. Biol. Med. Phys.* Vol. 4. New York: Academic Press.

Jones, I. H., and T. W. Meade (1964). Hypothermia following chlorpromazine therapy in myxoedematous patients. *Geront. Clin.* (Basel) 6:252-256.

Jones, K. (1955). *Lunacy, Law, and Conscience 1744-1845*. London: Routledge & Kegan Paul.

Jordan, M., M. Kepes, R. B. Hayes, and W. Hammond (1954). Dietary habits of persons living alone. *Geriatrics* 9:230-232.

Joshua, J. O. (1974). Responsible pet ownership. In R. S. Anderson, ed., *Pet Animals and Society*. Baltimore: Williams and Wilkins.

Kallmann, F. J. and G. Sander (1949). Twin studies on aging and longevity. *J. Hered.* 39:349-357.

Kannel, W. B., W. P. Castelli, and T. Gordon (1979). Cholesterol in the prediction of atherosclerotic disease. *Ann. Intern. Med.* 90:85-91.

Kannel, W. B., W. P. Castelli, T. Gordon, and P. M. McNamara (1971). Serum cholesterol, lipoproteins, and the risk of coronary heart disease — The Framingham Study. *Ann. Intern. Med.* 74:1-12.

Kannel, W. B., J. T. Doyle, D. T. Fredrickson, and W. R. Harlan (1978). Report of the Ad Hoc Committee on cigarette smoking and cardiovascular diseases for health professionals. Special report. *Circulation* 57:404a-405a.

Kannel, W. B., and T. Gordon, eds. (1969). *The Framingham Study. An Epidemiological Investigation of Cardiovascular Disease.* Serum cholesterol, systolic blood pressure and Framingham relative weight as discriminators of cardiovascular disease. Washington, DC: NIH-DHEW Report, Section 23.

Kaplan, H. S., and P. J. Tsuchitani, eds. (1978). *Cancer in China.* The report of the American Cancer Delegation visit to the People's Republic of China. New York: Alan R. Liss.

Katcher, A. (1979). Social support and health: Effects of pet ownership. *Proceedings of the Meeting of Group for the Study of Human/Companion Animal Bond.* Dundee, England. March 23-25.

Katz, L. N., and J. Stamler (1953). *Experimental Atherosclerosis.* Springfield, IL: Charles C. Thomas.

Katz, L. N., J. Stamler, and R. Pick (1958). *Nutrition and Atherosclerosis.* Philadelphia: Lea and Febiger.

Kavanau, J. L., J. Ramos, and R. M. Havenhill (1963). Compulsory regime and control of environment in animal behavior. I. Wheel running. *Behavior* 20: 251-281.

Kawakami, T. G., P. M. Buckley, A. DePaoli, W. Noll, and L. K. Bustad (1975). Studies on the prevalence of type C virus associated with gibbon hematopoietic neoplasms. In Y. Ito and R. M. Dutcher, eds., *Comparative Leukemia Research. Leukomogenesis.* Tokyo: University of Tokyo Press and Basel: S. Karger.

Kawakami, T. G., P. M. Buckley, and S. D. Huff (1972). Characterization of a C-type virus associated with gibbon lymphosarcoma. In E. I. Goldsmith and J. Moor-Jankowski, eds., *Medical Primatology (1972)* Part III. Basel: S. Karger.

Kawakami, T. G., P. M. Buckley, S. Huff, D. McKain, and H. Fielding (1973). A comparative study *in vitro* of a simian virus isolated from spontaneous woolly monkey fibrosarcoma and of a known feline fibrosarcoma virus. In R. M. Dutcher and L. Chieco-Bianchi, eds., *Unifying Concepts of Leukemia,* Basel: S. Karger.

Kearny, M. (1977). Pet therapy. *Animals* May/June:27-29.

Keddie, K. M. G. (1979). Problems associated with euthanasia of companion animals. *Proceedings of the Meeting of Group for the Study of the Human/Companion Animal Bond.* Dundee, England, March 23-25.

Kendall, M. J. (1979). Will drugs help patients with Alzheimer's disease? *Age Ageing* 8:86-92.

Keys, A. (1953). Atherosclerosis: A problem in newer public health. *J. Mt. Sinai Hosp.* 20:118-139.

Kibler, H. H., and H. D. Johnson (1966). Temperature and longevity in male rats. *J. Gerontol.* 21:52-56.

Kirkendall, M. (1973). Orman: The disabled pigeon who went to work. *Northwest Mag.* Sept. 2:12-13.

Klocke, R. A. (1977). Influence of aging on the lung. In C. E. Finch and L. Hayflick, eds., *Handbook of the Biology of Aging.* New York: Van Nostrand Reinhold.

Kobernick, S. D., G. Niwayama, and A. C. Zuchlewski (1957). Effect of physical activity on cholesterol atherosclerosis in rabbits. *Proc. Soc. Exp. Biol. Med.* 96:623-628.

Koehler, H. H., H. C. Lee, and M. Jacobson (1977). Tocopherols in canned entrees and vended sandwiches. *J. Am. Diet. Assoc.* 70:616-620.

Kohn, R. K. (1971) *Principles of Mammalian Aging.* Englewood Cliffs, N.J.: Prentice-Hall.

Kohn, R. R. (1977). Heart and cardiovascular system. In C. E. Finch and L. Hayflick, eds., *Handbook of the Biology of Aging.* New York: Van Nostrand Reinhold.

Kolata, G. B. (1979). Mental disorders: A new approach to treatment? *Science* 203:36-38.

Kottke, B. A. and M. T. R. Subbiah (1978). Pathogenesis of atherosclerosis. Concepts based on animal models. *Mayo Clin. Proc.* 53:35-48.

Kramer, J. W. (1977). Inherited early onset canine diabetes mellitus—a new model of human diabetes mellitus. *Fed. Proc.* 36:279.

Kritchevsky, D. (1974). Laboratory models for atherosclerosis. *Adv. Drug. Res.* 9: 41-53.

——— (1978). How aging affects cholesterol metabolism. *Postgrad Med.* 63(3):133-138.

Kruisbeek, A. M. (1978). *Thymus Dependent Immune Competence.* Rijswijk, The Netherlands: Institute of Experimental Gerontology of the Organization for Health Research, TNO.

Kumar, V. (1979). Diseases of Immunity. In S. D. Robbins and R. S. Cotran, eds., *Pathologic Basis of Disease.* Philadelphia: W. B. Saunders.

Kummerow, F. A., Y. Kim, M. D. Hull, J. Pollard, P. Illinov, D. L. Dorossien, and J. Valek (1977). The influence of egg consumption on the serum of cholesterol level in human subjects. *Am. J. Clin. Nutr.* 30:664-673.

Labouvie-Vief, G. (1979). *Does Intelligence Decline with Age?* Washington, DC: Government Printing Office, NIH Publication No. 79-1859.

Lacey, J. I., J. Kagen, B. C. Lacey, and H. A. Moss (1963). Situational determinants and behavioral correlates of automatic response patterns. In P. J. Knapp, ed., *Expression of the Emotions in Man.* New York: International University Press.

Lansing, A. I. (1952). General physiology. In A. I. Lansing, ed., *Cowdry's Problems of Aging.* Baltimore: Williams and Wilkins.

Leathers, C. W., M. G. Bond, and L. L. Rudel (1978). Effects of ethanol on dyslipoproteinemia and coronary artery atherosclerosis in nonhuman primates. *Circulation* 58 (Suppl 4):77

Leavitt, E. S. (1968). Animals and their legal rights. New York: *Animal Welfare Inst.* 44:165.

Lebeau, A. (1970). Dog and man—comparison of ages. *J. Am. Vet. Med. Assoc.* 157:1335.

Lee, J. C., L. M. Karpeles, and S. E. Downing (1972). Age-related changes of cardiac performance in male rats. *Am. J. Physiol* 222:432-438.

Lei, K. Y., and L. C. Yong (1979). Mineral content of bone and other tissues. In D. M. Bowden, ed., *Aging in Nonhuman Primates.* New York: Van Nostrand Reinhold.

Lesser, G. T., S. Deutsch, and J. Markofsky (1973). Aging in the rat: Longitudinal and cross-sectional studies of body composition. *Am. J. Physiol* 255:1472-1478.

Levinson, B. M. (1961). The dog as a "co-therapist." *Mental Hyg.* 46:59-65.

—— (1966). Pets: A special technique in child psychotherapy. *Nat. Humane Rev.* July-Aug.:24-27.

—— (1968). Interpersonal relationships between pet and human being. In M. W. Fox, ed., *Abnormal Behavior in Animals.* Philadelphia: Saunders.

—— (1969a). *Pet-oriented Child Psychotherapy.* Springfield, IL: Charles C. Thomas.

—— (1969b). Pets and old age. *Mental Hyg.* 53:364-368.

—— (1970). Nursing home pets: A psychological adventure for the patient. *Nat. Humane Rev.* July-Aug.:14-16 and Sept.-Oct.:6-8.

—— (1972). *Pets and Human Development.* Springfield, IL: Charles C. Thomas.

—— (1974). Pets and environment. In R. S. Anderson, ed., *Pet Animals and Society.* Baltimore: Williams and Wilkins.

Lew, E. A. (1959). *Build and Blood Pressure Study,* Vols. 1 and 2. Chicago: Society of Actuaries.

Lewis, C. S., ed. (1946). *George Macdonald Anthology.* London: Geoffrey Bles.

Libow, L. S. (1963). Medical investigation of the process of aging. In J. E. Biren, M. R. Yarrow, and S. W. Greenhouse, eds., *Human Aging: A Biological and Behavioral Study,* Chapter 5. Washington, DC: U.S. Government Printing Office.

Liebow, A. A. (1964). Biochemical and structural changes in the aging lung. Summary. In L. Cander and J. H. Moyer, eds., *Aging of the Lung.* New York: Grune and Stratton.

Lofland, H. B., Jr., T. B. Clarkson, and B. C. Bullock (1970). Whole body sterol metabolism in squirrel monkeys. *Exp. Mol. Pathol* 13:1-11.

Lorenz, K. Z. (1953). *Man Meets Dog.* New York: Penguin Books.

Luginbuhl, H. (1966). Spontaneous atherosclerosis in swine. In L. K. Bustad and R. O. McClellan, eds., *Swine in Biomedical Research.* Seattle: Frayn Printing.

Lutwak, L., L. Krook, P. A. Henrikson, R. Uris, J. Whalen, A. Coulston, and G. Lesser (1971). Calcium deficiency and human periodontal disease. *Isr. J. Med. Sci.* 7:504-505.

Lynch, J. J., G. F. Fregin, J. B. Mackie, and R. R. Monroe (1974). The effect of human contact on the heart activity of the horse. *Psychophysiology* 11:472-478.

Lynch, J. J., and J. F. McCarthy (1967). The effect of petting on a classically conditioned emotional response. *Behav. Res. Ther.* 5:55-62.

Lynch, J. J., and J. F. McCarthy (1969). Social responding in dogs: Heart rate changes to a person. *Psychophysiology* 5:389-393.

Lyons, J. S., and M. F. Trulson (1956). Food practices of older people living at home. *J. Gerontol* 11:66-72.

Lytle, L. D., and A. Altar (1979). Diet, central nervous system and aging. *Fed. Proc.* 38:2017-2022.

Maaske, C. A., N. H. Booth, and T. W. Nielsen (1966). Experimental right heart failure in swine. In L. K. Bustad and R. O. McClellan, eds., *Swine in Biomedical Research.* Seattle: Frayn Printing.

MacMillan, A. L., J. L. Corbett, R. H. Johnson, A. Crampton Smith, J. M. K. Spalding, and L. Wollner (1967). Temperature regulation in survivors of accidental hypothermia of the elderly. *Lancet* 2:165-169.

Magee, P. N., and J. M. Barnes (1956). The production of malignant primary hepatic tumors in the rat by feeding dimethylnitrosamine. *Br. J. Cancer* 10: 114-122.

——— (1967). Carcinogenic nitroso compounds. *Adv. Cancer Res.* 10:163-246.

Mahley, R. W., T. L. Inneravity, T. P. Bensot, A. Lipson, and S. Margolis (1978). Alterations in human high density lipoproteins with or without increased plasma-cholesterol, induced by diets high in cholesterol. *Lancet* 2:807-809.

Makinodan, T. (1978). The thymus in aging. In R. B. Greenblat, ed., *Geriatric Endocrinology* 5:217-230. New York: Raven Press.

Malinov, M. R., P. McLaughlin, L. Papworth, H. K. Naito, and L. A. Lewis (1976). Effect of bran and cholestyramine on plasma lipids in monkeys. *Am. J. Clin. Nutr.* 29:905-911.

Marx, J. L. (1979). The HDL: The good cholesterol carriers? *Science* 205:677-679.

Masoro, E. J. (1976). Physiologic changes with aging. In M. Winick, ed., *Nutrition and Aging.* New York: John Wiley and Sons.

Masoro, E. J., H. Bertrand, G. Liepa, and B. P. Yu (1979). Analysis and exploration of age-related changes in mammalian structure and function. *Fed. Proc.* 38: 1956-1961.

Mauderly, J. L. (1979). Effect of age on pulmonary structure and function of immature and adult animals and man. *Fed. Proc.* 38:173-177.

Maugh, T. H., II (1979). Cancer and environment: Higginson speaks out. *Science* 205:1363-1364, 1366.

May, S. H. (1958). The role of caloric intake and output balance in atherogenesis. *Am. J. Cardiol.* 2:1-4.

Mayer, J. (1974). Aging and nutrition. *Geriatrics* 29:57-59.

McCay, C. M., M. F. Crowell, and L. A. Maynard (1935). The effect of retarded growth upon the length of life span and upon the ultimate body size. *J. Nutr.* 10:63-79.

McCulloch, M. J. (1976). Contributions to Mental Health. In R. K. Anderson, ed., *A Description of the Responsibilities of Veterinarians as they Relate Directly to Human Health.* A report prepared for the Bureau of Health Manpower, U.S. DHEW, Contract 231-76-0202.

——— (1977). The veterinarian and human health care systems: Issues and boundaries. In L. B. McCullough and J. P. Morris III, eds., *Implications of History and Ethics to Medicine, Veterinary and Human.* Texas A&M University, College Station, TX: Centennial Academic Assembly.

——— (1979). Education programme methods for teaching pet owner relationships to health professionals. *Proceedings of Meeting of Group for the Study of Human/Companion Animal Bond.* Dundee, England, March 23-25.

Medawar, P. B. (1957). *The Uniqueness of the Individual.* London: Methuen.

Meek, E. S. (1977). Do persistent viral infections have a role in aging? *Geriatrics* 32(3):116-118, 121.

Messent, P. (1979). Behavioral patterns of companion animals—their significance in pet/owner bonding. *Proceedings of Meeting of Group for the Study of Human/Companion Animal Bond.* Dundee, England, March 23-25.

Metchnikoff, E. (1907). *The Prolongation of Life-Optimistic Studies.* London: Heinemann. As cited by Comfort (1956).

Meyer, W. H. (1979). Further comments. *Fed. Proc.* 38:2436-2437.

Meyers, K. M., H. Holmsen, C. L. Seachord, G. E. Hopkins, R. E. Borchard, and G. A. Padgett (1979a). Storage pool deficiency in platelets from Chediak-Higashi cattle. *Am. J. Physiol.* 237:239-248.

Meyers, K. M., C. L. Seachord, H. Holmsen, J. B. Smith, and D. J. Prieur (1979b). A dominant role of thromboxane formation in secondary aggregation of platelets. *Nature* 282:331-333.

Miller, D. S., and P. R. Payne (1968). Longevity and protein uptake. *Exp. Gerontol.* 3:231-234.

Miller, G. J., and N. E. Miller (1975). Plasma-high-density-lipoprotein concentration and development of ischemic heart-disease. *Lancet* 1:16-19.

Miller, J. A. (1973). Naturally occurring substances that can cause tumors. In *Toxicants Occurring Naturally in Foods.* 2nd ed. Washington, DC: National Academy of Sciences.

Miller, J. A., and E. C. Miller (1953). The carcinogenic aminoazo dyes. *Adv. Cancer Res.* 1:339-396.

—— (1976). Carcinogens occurring naturally in foods. *Fed. Proc.* 35(6):1316-1321.

Minnesota Humane Society (1972). Pets by prescription—a novel program of Minnesota Humane Society. *J. Am. Vet. Med. Assoc.* 161:971-972.

Moment, G. B. (1978). The Ponce de Leon trail today. In J. A. Behnke, C. E. Finch, and G. B. Moment, eds., *The Biology of Aging.* New York: Plenum Press.

Montagna, W. (1976). *Nonhuman Primates in Biomedical Research.* Minneapolis: University of Minnesota Press.

Moore, D. H., II (1975). A study of age group track and field records to relate age and running speed. *Nature* 253:264-265.

Morris, J. N., and J. A. Heady (1953). Mortality in relation to the physical activity of work. *Br. J. Ind. Med.* 10:245-254.

Morris, J. N., and M. D. Crawford (1958). Coronary heart disease and physical activity of work: Evidence of a national necropsy survey. *Br. Med. J.* 1:1485-1496.

Morris, J. N., J. A. Heady, and P. A. B. Raffle (1956). Epidemiology of uniforms. *Lancet* 271:569-570.

Mugford, R. (1979a). Basis of the normal and abnormal pet/owner bond. *Proceedings of Meeting of Group for the Study of Human/Companion Animal Bond.* Dundee, England, March 23-25.

—— (1979b). The social significance of pet ownership. In S. A. Corson, ed., *Ethology and Non-verbal Communication in Mental Health.* London: Pergamon Press.

Mugford, R. A., and J. G. M'Comisky (1975). Some recent work on the psychotherapeutic value of cage birds with old people. In R. S. Anderson, ed., *Pet Animals and Society*. Baltimore: Williams and Wilkins.

Muller, H. J. (1951). Strahlenschadigung des genetischen materials. *Strahlentherapie* 85:362-390.

Munoz, J. M., H. H. Sandstead, R. A. Jacob, G. M. Logan, Jr., S. J. Reck, L. M. Klevay, F. R. Dintzis, G. E. Inglett, and W. C. Shuey (1979). Effects of some cereal brans and textured vegetable protein on plasma lipids. *Am. J. Clin. Nutr.* 32:580-592.

Munro, H. N., and V. R. Young (1978). Protein metabolism in the elderly. *Postgrad. Med.* 63(3):143-152.

Myasnikov, A. L. (1958). Influence of some factors on development of experimental cholesterol atherosclerosis. *Circulation* 17:99-113.

National Academy of Sciences (1973). *Toxicants Occurring Naturally in Foods*. 2nd ed. Committee on Food Protection, Food and Nutrition Board, National Research Council, Washington, DC.

Newberne, P. M. (1965). Carcinogenicity of aflotoxin-contaminated peanut meal. In G. N. Wogan, ed., *Mycotoxins in Foodstuffs*. Cambridge, MA: M.I.T. Press.

Nichols, A. B., C. Ravenscroft, D. E. Lamphiear, and L. D. Ostrander (1976). Daily nutritional intake and serum lipid levels. The Tecumseh study. *Am. J. Clin. Nutr.* 29:1384-1392.

Novak, L. P. (1972). Aging, total body potassium, fat-free mass in males and females between ages 18-85 years. *J. Gerontol.* 27:438-443.

Oldstone, M. B. A., and F. J. Dixon (1974). Aging and chronic virus infection: Is there a relationship? *Fed. Proc.* 33:2057-2059.

Orma, E. J. (1957). Effect of physical activity on atherogenesis. An experimental study in cockerels. *Acta Physiol. Scand.* 41:supplement 142.

Osborne, T. B., L. B. Mendel, and E. L. Ferry (1917). The effect of retardation of growth upon breeding period and duration of life of rats. *Science* 45:294-295.

Ottenstein, D. M., L. A. Wittings, G. Walker, V. Mahadevan, and N. Pelick (1977). Trans fatty acid content of commercial margarine samples determined by gas liquid chromatography on OV-275. *J. Am. Oil Chem. Soc.* 54:207-209.

Paffenbarger, R. S., and W. E. Hale (1975). Work activity and coronary heart mortality. *N. Engl. J. Med.* 292:545-550.

Pearl, R. (1928). *The Rate of Living*. New York: Knopf.

Pelcovits, J. (1972). Nutrition to meet the human needs of older Americans. *J. Am. Diet Assoc.* 60:297-300.

Perryman, L. E. (1979). Primary and secondary immune deficiencies of domestic animals. *Adv. Vet. Sci. Comp. Med.* 23:23-52.

Pfaffenberger, C. J., J. P. Scott, J. L. Fuller, B. E. Ginsburg, and S. W. Bielfelt (1976). *Guide Dogs for the Blind: Their Selection, Development, and Training*. Amsterdam: Elsevier Scientific Publishing.

Pitot, H. C. (1977). Carcinogenesis and aging—two related phenomena? A review. *Am. J. Pathol.* 87:444-472.

Plum, F. (1979). Dementia: An approaching epidemic. *Nature* 279:372-373.

Pollock, G. A. (1979). Health risks from environmental contaminants. II. Pesticides and Mycotoxins. Presented at Am. Vet. Med. Assoc. convention, Seattle, July.

Porter, M. W., W. Yamanaka, S. D. Carlson, and M. A. Flynn (1977). Effect of dietary egg on serum cholesterol and triglyceride of human males. *Am. J. Clin. Nutr.* 30:490-495.

Posner, B. M. (1979). *Nutrition and the Elderly.* Lexington Books, Lexington, MA: D. C. Heath.

Prichard, R. W. (1974). Recent advances in molecular pathology: Regression of atherosclerosis—a perspective. *Exp. Mol. Pathol.* 20:407-411.

Prinz, P. N., and M. Raskind (1978). Aging and sleep disorders. In R. L. Williams and I. Karacan, eds., *Sleep Disorders. Diagnosis and Treatment.* New York: John Wiley and Sons.

Rao, D. B. (1973). Problems of nutrition in the aged. *J. Am. Geriatrics Soc.* 21: 362-367.

Rapacz, J., C. E. Elson, and J. J. Lalich (1977). Correlation of an immunogenetically defined lipoprotein type with aortic intimal lipidosis in swine. *Exp. Mol. Pathol.* 27:249-261.

Rapp, F. and C. L. Reed (1977). The viral etiology of cancer. *Cancer* 40:419-429.

Redmond, D. E. (1970). Tobacco and cancer: The first clinical report, 1761. *N. Engl. J. Med.* 282:18-23.

Reichel, W. (1978). The evaluation of the confused, disoriented or demented elderly patient. In W. Reichel, ed., *Clinical Aspects of Aging.* Baltimore: Williams and Wilkins.

Renold, A. E., A. E. Ganet, W. Stautfacher, and B. Jean-renaud (1968). Laboratory animals with spontaneous diabetes and/or obesity: Suggested suitability for the study of spontaneous atherosclerosis. *Prog. Biochem. Pharmacol.* 4:363-367.

Rizek, R. L., B. Friend, and L. Page (1974). Fat in today's food supply—level of use and sources. *J. Am. Oil Chem. Soc.* 51:244-250.

Robinson, D. (1980). Old people who jump for joy. *Parade* Feb. 3:23-25.

Robinson, M. H. (1977). On sugar and white flour . . . the dangerous twins. In R. J. Williams and D. K. Kalita, eds., *A Physician's Handbook on Orthomolecular Medicine.* New York: Pergamon Press.

Rockstein, M., and M. L. Sussman, eds. (1976). *Nutrition, Longevity and Aging.* New York: Academic Press.

Rockstein, M., M. L. Sussman, and J. Chesky, eds. (1974). *Theoretical Aspects of Aging.* New York: Academic Press.

Roffwarg, H. P., J. N. Muzio, and W. C. Dement (1966). Ontogenetic development of the human sleep-dream cycle. *Science* 152:604-619.

Rogers, A. E., and P. M. Newberne (1975). Dietary effects on chemical carcinogenesis in animal models for colon and liver tumors. *Cancer Res.* 35:3427-3431.

Ross, M. H. (1959). Protein, calories and life expectancy. *Fed. Proc.* 18:1190-1207.

—— (1976). Nutrition and longevity in experimental animals. In M. Winick, ed., *Nutrition and Aging.* New York: John Wiley and Sons.

—— (1978). Nutritional regulation of longevity. In J. A. Behnke, C. E. Finch, and G. B. Moment, eds., *The Biology of Aging.* New York: Plenum Press.

Ross, M. H., and G. Bras (1965). Tumor incidence patterns and nutrition in the rat. *J. Nutr.* 87:245-260.

—— (1974). Dietary preference and diseases of age. *Nature* 250:263-265.

Ross, R., and J. A. Glomset (1973). Atherosclerosis and the arterial smooth muscle cell. *Science* 180:1332-1339.

—— (1976). The pathogenesis of atherosclerosis (Pt. 1). *N. Engl. J. Med.* 295: 369-377.

Ross, R., and L. Harker (1976). Hyperlipidemia and atherosclerosis. *Science* 193: 1094-1100.

Ross, R., J. A. Glomset, B. Kariya, and L. A. Harker (1974). A platelet-dependent serum factor that stimulates the proliferation of arterial smooth muscle cells in vitro. *Proc. Natl. Acad. Sci.* 71:1207-1210.

Rous, P. (1911). A sarcoma of the fowl transmissible by an agent separable from the tumor cells. *J. Exp. Med.* 13:397-411.

—— (1965). Viruses and tumor causation. An appraisal of present knowledge. *Nature* 207:457-463.

Rowsell, H. C., J. F. Mustard, M. A. Packham, and W. J. Dodds (1966). The hemostatic mechanism and its role in cardiovascular disease of swine. In L. K. Bustad and R. O. McClellan, eds., *Swine in Biomedical Research.* Seattle: Frayn Printing.

Rubner, M. (1908). Das Problem der Lebensdauer und seine Beziehungen zu Wachstum und Ernahrung. Munich: R. Oldenbourg.

Rusch, H. P. (1944). Extrinsic factors that influence carcinogenesis. *Physiol. Rev.* 24:177-204.

Rynearson, E. K. (1978). Humans and pets and attachment. *Br. J. Psychiat.* 133: 550-555.

Sacher, G. A. (1956). On the statistical nature of mortality with especial reference to chronic radiation mortality. *Radiology* 67:250-257.

—— (1977). Life table modification and life prolongation. In C. E. Finch and L. Hayflick, eds., *Handbook of the Biology of Aging.* New York: Van Nostrand Reinhold.

Sacher, G. A., and P. H. Duffy (1979). Genetic relation of life span to metabolic rate for inbred mouse strains and their hybrids. *Fed. Proc.* 38:184-188.

Sanders, M., F. C. White, and C. M. Bloor (1977). Cardiovascular responses of dogs and pigs exposed to similar physiologic stress. *Comp. Biochem. Physiol.* 58a: 365-370.

Sanders, M., F. C. White, T. M. Peterson, and C. M. Bloor (1978). Effects of endurance exercise on coronary collateral blood flow in miniature swine. *Am. J. Physiol.* 234:H614-H619.

Sandstead, H. H., L. M. Klevay, R. A. Jacob, J. M. Munoz, G. M. Logan, Jr., S. J. Reck, F. R. Dintzis, G. E. Inglett, and W. C. Shuey (1979). Effects of dietary fiber and protein level on minimal element metabolism. In G. E. Inglett and S. I. Falkehag, eds., *Dietary Fibers: Chemistry and Nutrition.* New York: Academic Press.

Sandstead, H. H., J. M. Munoz, R. A. Jacob, L. M. Klevay, S. J. Reck, G. M. Logan, F. R. Dintzis, G. E. Inglett, and W. C. Shuey (1978). Influence of dietary fiber on trace element balance. *Am. J. Clin. Nutr.* 31:5180-5184.

Sassin, J. F., D. C. Parker, J. W. Mace, R. W. Gotlin, L. C. Johnson, and L. G. Rossman (1969). Human growth hormone release: Relation to slow wave sleep and sleep-waking cycles. *Science* 165:513-515.

Scheel, L. D. (1973). *Photosensitizing Agents in Toxicants Occurring Naturally in Foods.* 2nd ed. Washington DC: National Academy of Sciences.

Schiffman, S. (1977). Food recognition by the elderly. *J. Gerontol.* 32:586-592.

—— (1979). Changes in taste with age: Psychophysical aspects. In J. M. Ordy and K. R. Brizzie, eds., *Sensory Systems and Communication in the Elderly*. Aging, Vol. 10. New York: Raven Press.

Schwabe, C. W. (1978). *Cattle, Priests, and Progress in Medicine*. Minneapolis: University of Minnesota Press.

Scott, J. P. (1962). Critical periods in behavioral development. *Science* 138:949-958.

Scott, J. P., and J. L. Fuller (1950). *Manual of Dog Testing Techniques*. Bar Harbor, Maine: Roscoe B. Jackson Memorial Laboratory.

—— (1965). *Genetics and the Social Behavior of the Dog*. Chicago: University of Chicago Press.

Shefer, V. F. (1973). Absolute number of neurons and thickness of cerebral cortex during aging, senile and vascular dementia and Pick's and Alzheimer's Disease. *Neurosci. Behav. Physiol.* 6:319-324.

Shelanski, M. L. (1975). The aging brain: Alzheimers disease and senile dementia. In A. M. Ostfeld and D. C. Gibson, eds., *Epidemiology of Aging*. Bethesda, MD: U.S. DHEW Publication No. (NIH) 75-711.

Shephard, R. J. (1978). Exercise and aging. In J. A. Behnke, C. E. Finch, and G. B. Moment, eds., *The Biology of Aging*, New York: Plenum Press.

Shock, N. W. (1960). Discussion on mortality and measurement. In B. L. Strehler, J. D. Ebert, H. B. Glass, and N. W. Shock, eds., *The Biology of Aging: A Symposium*. Washington, DC: American Institute of Biological Sciences.

—— (1962). The science of gerontology. In E. C. Jeffers, ed., *Proc. Seminars 1959-1961 Durham, NC Council on Gerontology*. Durham: Duke University Press.

—— (1970). Physiologic aspects of aging. *J. Am. Diet. Assoc.* 56:491-496.

—— (1974). Physiological theories of aging. In M. Rockstein, M. Sussman, and J. Chesky, eds., *Theoretical Aspects of Aging*. New York: Academic Press.

—— (1977). Systems integration. In C. E. Finch and L. Hayflick, eds., *Handbook of the Biology of Aging*. New York: Van Nostrand Reinhold.

—— (1979). Systems physiology and aging. *Fed. Proc.* 38:161-162.

Shock, N. W., and A. H. Norris (1970). Physical activity and aging. In D. Brunner and E. Jokl, eds., *Med. and Sport*. Basel: S. Karger. 4:92-99.

Siegal, J. S. (1975). Some demographic aspects of aging in the United States. Bethesda, MD: DHEW Publicaton No. (NIH) 75-711.

Siegel, A. (1962). Reaching severely withdrawn through pet therapy. *Am. J. Psychiatry* 118:1045-1046.

Sigurdsson, B. R. (1954). A chronic encephalitis of sheep with general remarks on infections which develop slowly, and some of their special characteristics. *Br. Vet. J.* 110:341-354.

Silverberg, E. (1979). Cancer statistics, 1979. *CA.* 29(1):6-21.

Simons, M. A. P. (1974). The horse as a friend of man: Its value and future. In R. S. Anderson, ed., *Pet Animals and Society*. Baltimore: Williams and Wilkins.

Sirtori, C., G. Ricci, and S. Gorini, eds. (1973). *Diet and Atherosclerosis*. New York: Plenum Press.

Slack, J. (1969). Risks of ischemic heart-disease in familial hyperlipoprotein-aenemic states. *Lancet* 2:1380-1382.

Slack, J., and N. C. Nevin (1968). Hyperlipidaemic xanthomatoses. 1) Increased risk of death from ischaemic heart disease in first degree relatives of 53 patients with essential hyperlipidaenemia and xanthomatosis. *J. Med. Genet.* 5:4-8.

Smith, R. W., and J. Rizek (1966). Epidemiologic studies of osteoporosis in women of Puerto Rico and southeastern Michigan with special reference to age, race, national origin, and to other related or associated findings. *Clin. Orthop.* 45: 31-48.

Smithcors, J. F. (1959). Veterinariana. *Mod. Vet. Pract.* Dec. 15.

Snyder, S. P., and G. H. Theilen (1969). Transmissible feline fibrosarcoma. *Nature* 221:1074-1075.

Sokolow, M., and M. B. McIlroy (1979) *Clinical Cardiology.* 2nd ed. Los Altos, Calif: Lange Medical Publications.

Solon, J. A. (1978). Alternative models of physician leadership in long-term care facilities. In W. Reichel, ed., *Clinical Aspects of Aging.* Baltimore: Williams and Wilkins.

Spencer, G. R. (1979). Osteoporosis. *Am. J. Pathol.* 95:277-280.

Spink, W. W. (1979). *Infectious Diseases. Prevention and Treatment in the Nineteenth and Twentieth Centuries.* Minneapolis: University of Minnesota Press.

Stamler, J. (1975). Diet-related risk factors for human atherosclerosis: Hyperlipidemia, hypertension, hyperglycemia—current status. *Adv. Exp. Med. Biol.* 60:125-158.

Stout, R. W. (1979). Three views on geriatric medicine: 1) Hospital care of the elderly: General or geriatric medicine. *Age Ageing* 8(3):137-140.

Strehler, B. L. (1977). *Time, Cells and Aging.* 2nd ed. New York: Academic Press.

Stunkard, A. J. (1976). Nutrition, aging and obesity. In M. Rockstein and M. L. Sussman, eds., *Nutrition, Longevity, and Aging.* New York: Academic Press.

Succec, A. (1969). Oxygen uptake and heart rate in middle-aged males participating in an adult fitness program. *Am. Correct. Therap. J.* 23:98-103.

Sweatman, T. W. and A. G. Renwick (1979). Saccharin metabolism and tumorgenicity. *Science* 205:1019.

Takahashi, Y., D. M. Kipnis, and W. H. Daughaday (1968). Growth hormone secretion during sleep. *J. Clin. Invest.* 47:2079-2094.

Tannenbaum, A. (1942). The genesis and growth of tumors. III. Effects of a high-fat diet. *Cancer Res.* 2:468-475.

Tannenbaum, A., and H. Silverstone (1953). Nutrition in relation to cancer. *Adv. Cancer Res.* 1:452-501.

Theilen, G. H., D. Gould, M. Fowler, and D. Dungworth (1971). C-type virus tumor tissue of a woolly monkey (*Lagothrix* spp.) with a fibrosarcoma. *J. Natl. Cancer Inst.* 47:881-889.

Thorbecke, G. J., ed. (1975). *Biology of Aging and Development.* New York: Plenum Press.

Timiras, P. S. (1978). Biological perspectives on aging. *Am. Scient.* 66:605-613.

Timiras, P. S., and A. Bignami (1976). Pathology of the aging brain. In M. F. Elias, B. E. Eleftheriou, and P. K. Elias, eds., *Special Review of Experimental Aging Research, Progress in Biology.* Bar Harbor: EAR.

Todhunter, E. N., and W. J. Darby (1978). Guidelines for maintaining adequate nutrition in old age. *Geriatrics* 33(6):49-56.

Trew, C. G. (1949). *The Story of the Dog and His Uses to Mankind.* New York: E. P. Dutton.

Truswell, A. S. (1978). Diet and plasma lipids—a reappraisal. *Am. J. Clin. Nutr.* 31:977-989.

Tzankoff, S. P., S. Robinson, F. S. Pyke, and C. A. Brawn (1972). Physiological adjustments to work in older men as affected by physical training. *J. Appl. Physiol.* 33:346-350.

Urist, M. R. (1960). Cage layer osteoporosis. *Endocrinol.* 67:879-880.

—— (1971). Osteoporosis in post-menopausal women. *The Medical Folio.* 3(3). New York: Wilson Research Foundation.

—— (1973a). Orthopaedic management of osteoporosis in postmenopausal women. *Clinics in Endocrinology and Metabolism.* 2:159-186.

—— (1973b). Osteoporosis versus osteomalacia: Diagnosis and management in postmenopausal women. In *Instructional Course Lectures: The American Academy of Orthopedic Surgeons.* 13:1-11. St. Louis: C. V. Mosby.

Veatch, R. M. (1979). *Life Span: Values and Life-Extending Technologies.* San Francisco: Harper and Row.

Vesselinovitch, D. (1979). Animal modes of atherosclerosis, their contributions and pitfalls. *Artery* 5:193-206.

Vesselinovitch, D., R. W. Wissler, K. Fisher-Dzoga, R. Hughes, and L. Dubien (1974). Regression of atherosclerosis in rabbits. Treatment with low-fat diet, hyperoxia and hypolipidemic agents. *Atherosclerosis* 19:259-275.

Voith, V. L. (1979). Clinical animal behavior. *Calif. Vet.* 33(6):21-25.

Vollmer, P. J. (1977) The new puppy: Preventing problems through thoughtful selection. *Vet. Med. Small Anim. Clin.* December: 1823-1824.

—— (1978). The new puppy 2: Preventing problems through thoughtful selection. *Vet. Med. Small Anim. Clin.* Jan.: 31-32.

Walford, R. L. (1969). *The Immunological Theory of Aging.* Copenhagen: Munksgaard.

Walford, R. L., R. K. Liu, M. Mathies, M. Gerbase-Delima, and L. Lipps (1974). Longterm dietary restriction and immune function in mice, response to sheep red blood cells and to mitogens. *Mech. Age. Dev.* 2:447-450.

Walker, A. R. P. (1975). Effect of high crude fiber intake on transit times and the absorption of nutrients in South African negro school children. *Am. J. Clin. Nutr.* 28:1161-1169.

Wallin, P. (1978). Pets and mental health: Some psychological perspectives on the pet/person relationship and implications for veterinary practice. In *The Newer Knowledge About Dogs.* 28th Gaines Veterinary Symposium, Tuskegee Institute, Alabama.

Walster, D. (1979). The role of pets in the mental health of the elderly. *Proceedings of Meeting of Group for the Study of Human/Companion Animal Bond.* Dundee, England, March 23-25.

Watkin, D. M. (1973). Nutrition for the aging and the aged. In R. S. Goodhart and M. E. Shils, eds., *Modern Nutrition in Health and Disease.* 5th ed. Philadelphia: Lea and Febiger.

Weg, R. B. (1978). *Nutrition and the Later Years.* Los Angeles: University of Southern California Press.

Weir, D. R., H. B. Houser, M. Davis, and E. Schenk (1978). Recognition and management of the nutrition problems of the elderly. In W. Reichel, ed., *Clinical Aspects of Aging.* Baltimore: Williams and Wilkins.

Weyman, A. E., D. M. Greenbaum, and W. J. Grace (1974). Accidental hypothermia in an alcoholic population. *Am. J. Med.* 56:13-21.

White, J. W., Jr. (1975). Relative significance of dietary sources of nitrate and nitrite. *J. Agric. Food Chem.* 23:886-891.

White, P. D. (1958). Safe bicycling. *N. Engl. J. Med.* 259:499-500.

Whitney, L. F. (1971). *Dog Psychology.* New York: Howell Book House.

Widdowson, E. M., and G. C. Kennedy (1962). Rate of growth, mature weight and life span. *Proc. Roy. Soc. London., Series B, Biological Sciences* 156:96-108.

Wilbur, R. H. (1976). Pets, pet ownership and animal control: Social and psychological attitudes. In *Proceedings of the National Conference on Dog and Cat Control.* Denver, CO, Feb. 3-5.

Wilkie, F., and C. Eisdorfer (1971). Intelligence and blood pressure in the aged. *Science* 172:959-962.

Williams, C. (1971). Horsemanship for the handicapped. *West. Horseman* September:67-70.

Williams, R. J. (1956). *Biochemical Individuality.* New York: John Wiley and Sons.

Williamson, J. (1979). Three views on geriatric medicine: 3) Notes on the historical development of geriatric medicine as a medical specialty. *Age Ageing* 8:144-148.

Wilson, R. B., C. C. Middleton, and G. Y. Sun. (1978). Vitamin E, antioxidants and lipid peroxidation in experimental atherosclerosis of rabbits. *J. Nutr.* 108:1858-1867.

Wissler, R. W., and D. Vesselinovitch (1975). Regression of atherosclerosis in experimental animals and man. In *Verhandlunge der Deutschen gesellschaft fur innere medizin* 81:857-865.

Wolff, E. (1970). *A Survey of the Use of Animals in Psychotherapy in the United States.* Philadelphia:American Humane Association.

Wolff, I. A., and A. E. Wasserman (1972). Nitrates, nitrites and nitrosamines. *Science* 177:15-18.

Wolinsky, H. (1973). Mesenchymal response of the blood vessel wall. A potential avenue for understanding and treating atherosclerosis. *Circ. Res.* 32:543-549.

Wong, H. Y. C., S. N. David, S. O. Orimilikwe, and F. B. Johnson (1973). The effects of physical exercise in reversing experimental atherosclerosis. In C. Sirtori, G. Ricci, and S. Gorini, eds., *Diet and Atherosclerosis.* New York: Plenum Press.

Wong, H. Z., T. K. Greenfield, and J. A. Grubman (1977). *Index to the Substance Use and the College Experience Questionnaires 1974-1977.* Ann Arbor, MI: University of Michigan Counseling Services.

Wurtman, R. J. (1976). Control of brain neurotransmitter synthesis by precursor availability and nutritional state. *Biochem. Pharmacol.* 25:1691-1696.

Wynder, E. L., and B. S. Reddy (1975). Editorial: Dietary fat and colon cancer. *J. Natl. Cancer Inst.* 54:7-10.

Youmans, E. G., and M. Yarrow (1971). Aging and social adaptation: A longitudinal study of healthy old men. In S. Granieck and R. D. Patterson, eds., *Human Aging II: An Eleven Year Follow-up Biomedical and Behavioral Study*. DHEW publication No. HSM 70-9037. Washington, DC: U.S. Government Printing Office.

Yoxall, A., and M. Yoxall (1979). The multidisciplinary approach to pet/owner relationship problems. *Proceedings of Meeting of Group for the Study of Human/Companion Animal Bond*. Dundee, England, March 23-25.

Zanni, E., D. H. Calloway, and A. Y. Zezulka (1979). Protein requirements of elderly men. *J. Nutr.* 109: 513-524.

Index

INDEX

221

exercise, effect on, 175; expectancy,
iii, 71; extension, suggestions for,
49; and heredity, effect on, 39; and
lifestyle, effect on, 177; of mam-
mals, 12, 16; and metabolic rate,
effect on, 40; and protein in diet,
effect on, 34-35; of twins, 39. *See
also* Aging
Linoleic acid. *See* Fatty acids
Lipids, classification of, 102
Lithium, in combination choline to
treat mania, 111
Liver disease, and alcohol, 168
Llama, 5
Locomotion, deterioration with age.
See Aging
Loneliness, in elderly, 109, 111-12,
124, 169
Low density lipoprotein (LDL), 70
Lung function, aging changes in, 21-
22
Lymphosarcomas, in animals, 89

Malnutrition, 169
Margarine: saturated fat, 103; as substi-
tute for butter, 171
Masoro, Ed., 27, 34, 49
Massachusetts SPCA, 135
Mauderly, Joe, 21
Meat, as source of protein, 170
Medical curriculum, and needs of
elderly, iii, 113-14
Menning, Ed, 119
Mental disorders, in elderly, 59, 109-12,
168, 177
Mental hospitals, use of animals in, 4
Metabolism, 24. *See also* Aging
Milk, 172; pasteurization, 174; raw, as
cause of diseases, 174
Minerals, 172; as anticarcinogens, 106;
in taste and wound healing, 172
Models, animal. *See* Animal(s)
Mortality data, for animals and humans,
14-16, 50
Muscular strength, change with age,
27
Myocardial infarction, 122; survival
after, 123

National Academy of Sciences Food
and Nutrition Board, and recom-
mended dietary allowance, 168
Native Americans, and animals, 7
Natural foods, 173-74
Nervous system, changes with age, 29-
30
Neuroendocrine control, 48
Neurotransmitters, and aging, 48
Nicotine, effects on cardiovascular
function, 80
Nitrites and nitrates, 92-95
Nitrosamine, 93-95; inhibition by vita-
min C, 106
North American Riding for the Handi-
capped, 130
Nursing homes: animals in, 4; costs of,
iii
Nutrition, 59, 168

Obesity, 177
Oils. *See* Fats and oils
Olfactory acuity. *See* Aging
Osler, William, 56
Osteoporosis, 59, 107-9, 168, 177
Overeating, effect on health, 177

Partnerships of animals and humans, 6-
10
Pawling Convalescent Hospital, 118-19;
See also Animal-facilitated therapy
Pectin, as a source of fiber, 172
People-Pet Partnership at Washington
State University, 132-33, 137, 146
Periodontal disease, 59, 107-8, 177
Periodontitis, relation to osteoporosis,
108
Pet Animal Loan Service, 134
Pet banks, 134
Pet health plans, 166
Pet ownership, and survival, 123. *See
also* Animal(s); Animal-facilitated
therapy
Pet placement, 137-40; potential prob-
lems of, 162-65
Pet-a-Care, 133, 166
Phospholipids, fatty acid incorporation
in, 104